BEAST

A Slightly Irreverent Tale

About Cancer

(And Other Assorted Anecdotes)

APRIL 2014

THANK YOU FOR SUPPORTING

THE WAR AGAINST

THE BEAST!

BEST WISHES,

JAMES

THANK YOU FOR SUPPORTING

THE BEAST!

BEAST

A Slightly Irreverent Tale

About Cancer

(And Other Assorted Anecdotes)

James Capuano

2012
New Street Communications, LLC
Wickford, RI

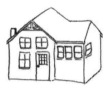

newstreetcommunications.com

Published 2012 by
New Street Communications, LLC
Wickford, Rhode Island
newstreetcommunications.com

Note: This book is not designed to provide medical advice. Medical explanations described here-in are not intended to be a substitute for professional medical advice, diagnosis or treatment. Never disregard professional medical advice, or delay in seeking it, because of something you have read in this volume or, for that matter, anywhere else.

Dedication

For Dana, Nick, Danny, Brandon and Jules; And for my Mother, who intuitively understood that kindness and laughter are the keys to the kingdom.

Contents

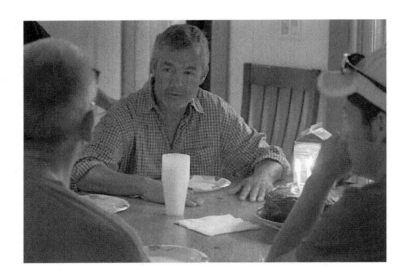

The author, Fire Island, 2012.

Preface

I know what you're thinking. I do. You're thinking: "Oh, God; not *another* book about cancer. If I wanna get depressed I'll look at my bank statement." Or, perchance it is a book along the lines of: "Oh, gee; isn't life so special and every minute so precious now that I've survived cancer?" *Please.*

I know that's what you're thinking and I don't blame you. Really. You're probably feeling a little bit bad about it too. No worries. This isn't one of *those* stories anyway. Yeah, sure — there's a whole bunch of stuff about cancer in here, but only because I happen to have been randomly selected to play host to that disgusting little cellular abnormality. Fear not my friends, as that's just part of the story. There's all kinds of other stuff in here as well.

I'd be lying, however, if I said that amid all the humorous anecdotes about loss of control, loyalty, honor, facing challenges, family values, parenthood, and unconditional friendship, I'm not trying to pass on some hard-earned knowledge about cancer diagnosis and treatment; about how when faced with the unimaginable you can't curl yourself up into a little ball and hope the scary monster will go away. Buck up. Take a deep breath, rear your head back and spit. Spit hard and spit angry. PUHH! It's amazing what we're capable of when our backs are to the wall and we're about to get slammed.

2

*

Please allow me to state the obvious (a task I have mastered after many years of Zen-like preparation): *Cancer sucks*. It will always suck. It especially sucks if you actually have it. We hate cancer. We even hate to say the word. And by "we," I mean those of us still living and breathing. It's as if by saying the word out loud we'll somehow catch it. Doctors don't even like to say it — they often refer to it simply as "the disease." We use hushed tones and speak in code: "He has you-know-what," "Yup, it's the Big C" — or, in the vernacular of my own doctor: "We also found some lesions on your small intestine." (Yikes! What the fuck is that supposed to mean? I thought a lesion was a cut of some sort.)

When we hear that someone we know has cancer, our immediate reaction is, "Oh boy, he's fucked." That's normal, I guess. It's been ingrained in our psyches for generations. "What the hell are *we* supposed to do about it?" you're probably asking yourself. My answer:

Attitude, my friends — attitude. And by *attitude* I don't mean powerless *hope* but rather plain old pissed-off "get the fuck out of my neighborhood" *attitude*.

I'd say *fighting attitude*, but that phrase is inadequate. This isn't just a fight. Fighting is schoolyard stuff. This is all-out war. Quite literally *do or die*. We need to go nuclear. Failure is not an option. We simply can't allow the bad-guy cells to win over the good-guy cells. We hate when that happens. We absolutely need for the good-guy cells to ride off into the sunset with the pretty girl cells and live happily ever after. Nice and tidy.

Don't get me wrong, I felt absolutely paralyzed when Dr. Keltner told me, "Well, it's Stage IV because it has spread to another organ" in answer to my insightful question: "What stage is it, doctor?" (For those of you who may not be up to speed on all the fancy cancer lingo, Stage IV is the one that takes you dangerously close to that last exit on life's highway— the one that alerts St. Peter to start scanning the ledger while King David dusts off the throne, Allah readies the vestal virgins, and Buddha oils up the Karmic wheel.)

But then the strangest thing happened. An eerie calm came over me and the paralysis started to melt away as I realized I wasn't scared. Dumbstruck maybe, shocked for sure, but not scared. I guess my subconscious was sending me subliminal messages telling me to relax; that it was better to know than to sit around wondering, lost in a haze of confusion and anxiety. Knowing was the first step toward staying alive. Knowing allowed me to focus on what I needed to do to help fix the problem. (You see, since Keltner was willing to take on the colossal task of conquering the beast in me called cancer, I figured the least I could do was help.) And perhaps by helping I made it possible for me to be here today, sharing my laudable little tale with you. Perhaps a bit more than "perhaps," actually. I mean, I battled the shit out of this thing. And it appears to be paying off.

But Enough About Cancer,
Let's Talk About Me

I grew up in New York City in the '60s and '70s, just about the best time in recorded history to be coming of age. The future was full of sex, drugs, and rock & roll. I lived in a huge apartment complex called Stuyvesant Town which, until recently, was privately owned and operated by the Metropolitan Life Insurance Company. Met Life built Stuy Town in the mid-1940s at a time when profit, greed, and "shareholder value" (a nicer way of saying "greed") were not yet the driving forces behind corporate America's existence. The place was actually built to provide returning World War II vets and civil servants (cops and firemen) with decent, affordable Manhattan housing. Very noble. Of course, all that has changed now, but growing up in that place at that time was a gift.

Stuyvesant Town is an 80-acre oasis in New York City that feels like a New England college campus: grass, trees, fountains, red brick buildings. It's bordered on the east by the aptly named East River, which separates Manhattan from Brooklyn and Queens; on the west by Gramercy Park, where I live now; on the south by the East Village (which sounds a bit confusing); and on the north by Kip's Bay and Murray Hill (don't know who Kip and Murray were, but they must have been important).

No matter how old you were, there were always a

hundred kids your age to hang out with. My particular group of friends was exceptionally clever and sarcastic. *Very* sarcastic. Couldn't be more brutal. It would usually start with one of us jumping all over some ill-advised thing another of us had said or done ("I don't wanna shoot hoops; I just took a shower and I don't feel like getting all sweaty"). Within moments, the whole gang was on the poor schmuck. ("Did you remember to put a tampon in after you douched, you little bitch?") It was all downhill from there. Best to shut up and go along for the ride, because no one could mount a formidable enough comeback to an onslaught of such magnitude.

It's exactly how we are with each other to this day whenever we get together, and I wouldn't want it any other way.

*

John Messina and I became friends in sixth grade when he transferred from St. Emerick's, a Catholic elementary school in the East Village, to the equally-Catholic Epiphany School in Gramercy Park, where many of my friends and I were learning how to be good little Christians. If you lived in the southern portion of Stuy Town and you were Catholic, you either went to St. Emerick's or the Immaculate Conception School; those of us on the northern end went to Epiphany.

I first noticed John on the way to school my first morning back after a long, lazy summer vacation in 1970. He was walking up ahead of me through the park on 20th Street with his mom. (We were beyond the boundaries of Stuyvesant Town at this point, so if you're picturing a lush, green park with grass and trees and benches with old people feeding pigeons and squirrels, erase that image and start over. Picture instead a slab of concrete roughly the size of half a city block, surrounded by a 20-foot-high chain-link fence, with four basketball hoops, and a baseball diamond painted on the cement.) Somehow I knew he and I were going to end up in the same class.

By this time I had already developed a reputation, rightly or wrongly, as a "tough" kid. I mention this because while walking behind John that fateful morning, rather than thinking normal thoughts, — like, "Gee, I wonder if he's nice," or "I wonder if he'll be in my class," I was sizing him up, trying to figure out whether or not I could "take" him. He was a pretty stocky kid and looked like he could fight. Not that any of us actually fought one another — it was more about posturing. I quickly decided I had the clear advantage, having already established myself over the past five years, whereas John was the new kid (even though lots of us already knew him from Stuy Town). It took all of two days, after realizing it wasn't worth the reputational risk of coming to blows, for us to establish a friendship that would carry us through the rest of our lives.

Our families grew close and we vacationed together. John and I even "lived" together for a brief period of time when we were seventeen. His maternal grandparents had an apartment in the same building as his parents.

He called one night while I was eating dinner with my family — breaded pork chops, the other white meat. (There was always meat on the menu. Italians are serious carnivores, and it just isn't a meal without the meat.) John and I were going to an Eagles concert at Madison Square Garden that night, and I figured he was calling to make plans to meet. John was renowned for making up ridiculous stories and doing ridiculous things, so of course I didn't believe him when he told me he couldn't go to the concert because his grandfather had been horribly murdered in the lobby of his building hours before.

"That's crossing the line, even for you," I said in disgust. "Why would you say something so horrendous?"

"Jimmy," he said, "I know I always say crazy things but I'm not joking around this time, my grandfather was killed today."

Well I have to tell you, that news really fucked up my evening. I wound up going to the concert anyway but I had a miserable time. After the funeral, John's grandmother, "Grandma Dolly," moved in with John's family, which left her apartment vacant for three weeks until her lease was due to expire. It didn't seem right to me, John, or our friend Chuck to just let that apartment sit empty when we could be in there hosting parties every night and acting like big-shots for the next three weeks.

It took some doing to convince our parents to let us move in: "Look, I'm going off to college in six months and this is a perfect opportunity for me to get a feel for what it's like living on my own."

My father was having none of it. "Stop talking to me like I'm a goddamned fool," Pops replied. "You just want to party with your idiot friends all night, so forget it."

My mother managed to talk him into it, and before long I was packing some clothes and moving away. Two minutes away, but still we had a ball, with parties and hordes of people in and out of the apartment, just as my dad had predicted, for three golden, glorious weeks. It was fantastic each night until it was time for bed, at which point John and I would slide into a panic, certain that his grandfather's ghost would show up to chastise us for all the bad things we had done in his apartment just hours before. There was only one bedroom and it had twin beds, so the three of us rotated sleeping in the beds and on the living room couch. Neither John nor I slept a wink whenever it was our turn on the couch because we were busy suffocating under the layers of blankets that were meant to shield us from the ghost of "Grandpa" Carillo. Chuck couldn't care less and slept like a rock, but John and I each kept one eye open waiting for the sun to rise, at which point we'd be safe again. What dopes.

Billy Smith and I go back a long way as well. Our families go back even longer. Our grandparents lived in the same building on 21st Street and First Avenue and were friends when they were newlyweds. My father grew up with Billy's uncle in that same building; and Billy, my brother and I carried on the tradition, growing up and hanging out together in Stuy Town. All in, we're talking about friendships that span over 80 years.

Billy, like me, had a reputation for being tough, only his was better deserved. His grandfather had him fighting in junior Golden Gloves boxing matches from the time he was strong enough to actually hold up the 16-ounce boxing gloves without falling over. (They were about the size of his head.)

One day in fifth grade, there was a commotion in the hall. Sister Thaddeus (the name alone was frightening; making matters worse, this "Sister of Charity" who was passing herself off as a "teacher" appeared to have *carte blanche* to lay hand upon us whenever she saw fit, and lay hand she did) proceeded to rip the door open just as Billy happened to be walking by, minding his own business. She pulled him into the classroom by his collar and simultaneously cracked him across the side of his head with an open hand (and no explanation whatsoever) in order, I suppose, to teach us all a little discipline, Roman Catholic style. The rest of us sat there in shock, thinking "Holy shit, she's fucking crazy," while Billy, who had no idea why he was getting beat up by a 50-year-old nun, cocked his arm, clenched his fist, and was ready to throw a left hook when he suddenly thought better of it. Instead, he apologized for doing nothing, and stood there, red-faced and humiliated.

Sister Thaddeus couldn't care less whether Billy was the real source of the commotion or not. She just needed to satisfy her deep-seated urge to smack the shit out of someone. I can only imagine what would have transpired had Billy actually thrown that punch. Probably a pack of nuns would have appeared out of nowhere and beat poor Billy to within an inch of his life.

It's obvious to me now that those nuns (in Sister Thaddeus' case, that was an acronym for *Not Unlike Nazis*) were part of some James Bond worship cult — dressing in what appeared to be the female version of a tuxedo, with that crazy little hat they tied under the chin. They were very clearly "licensed to kill." What a racket they had.

Then there's Tommy Dwyer. Tommy and I met in the first grade and have been through a lot together. We used to walk home for lunch every day in the sixth grade. (Amazingly, we were allowed to leave the school by ourselves at that tender age and wander the streets alone.) With about 45 minutes before we needed to be back in the classroom, we found all kinds of ways to get into trouble during the fifteen minutes it took to walk home and back, and we were almost always late, thereby extending our window of opportunity. We were instructed by our parents and the school principal in no uncertain terms to follow a designated route each way so as to avoid unnecessary conflict, which, in New York City in the early

'70s, we were fairly certain to run into.

There was one block they really warned us to stay away from: East 22nd Street, which accommodated a home for wayward inner-city youth (that's politically correct today-speak for what was more commonly referred to in the late '60s and early '70s as "tough black kids who got into trouble a lot"). They might as well have told us to avoid breathing oxygen. Once they made that pronouncement, it was a lock that we'd be walking down East 22nd Street all day, every day. Foolishly, Tommy and I enjoyed taunting the wayward inner-city youth as much as they enjoyed taunting us back, thankfully without serious consequence. "Too bad you suck," we'd yell as we flew by (we weren't very good at taunting yet).

One day as we were running by, they let loose with a pack of dogs, and the dogs would have had us had we not already been in full stride. We managed to jump onto the roof of a parked car moments before the hounds could sink their sharp little canines into us.

"Yeah, what was you sayin', white boy?" the kids taunted us. "We couldn't hear you 'cause-a all the barking."

The puppies held us at bay for the majority of the lunch period, forcing us to make up yet another story as to why we were late: "We ran into an old lady who was having trouble carrying her stuff so we helped her home and we felt bad leaving right away because she looked so lonely, and we think she was crying," we lied, angelically.

Lying was pretty easy to get away with in those days, as there were no cell phones and no reasonable ways to check out a story. Not that we wouldn't have helped a sobbing, lonely old lady had the need arisen. We were, after all, good little Christians.

Matty Warshaw was the outlier among us. In a sizable group of 95% Irish, 5% Italian and 100% Catholic kids, Matty was Jewish, of Russian descent. He lived up the block from Stuy Town and went to PS40, the local public school, and was adept at mixing with the Goyim. He played on our CYO sports teams, came to our parties, and at an early age went out with our "women." To this day, he maintains an inaccurate accounting of what transpired between him, Tara Keene and me when we were in the sixth grade.

It started when I concocted a plan to have John jokingly ask out a girl named Patty while I jokingly asked out Tara, with the intention of breaking up with them a day or two later. ("Going out" with a girl simply meant you agreed to be boyfriend and girlfriend in principle, which in no way obligated you to speak to or go near each other.) John went along with this, thinking it would be good for a laugh — even though he was madly in love with Marie Frey. What he didn't realize was that I actually *did* like Tara but didn't have the nerve to ask her out without this subterfuge.

After school one day, just before summer vacation, we set our plan in motion. It worked out great for me but created unimaginable grief for John. Patty was not one to take shit from anyone and she made John painfully aware of it in front of everyone: "You think that's funny, motherfucker? What are you, a fagot? I'll kick your fuckin' ass." I am not making this up. I was very much afraid of little Patty. The fact that she was way more sexually aware than the rest of us made her all the more terrifying.

Three weeks later, I was off with my family to the Catskill Mountains, where I fell head over heels for Alyson Bruu and instantly forgot that I ever even knew a girl named Tara Keene. (I know — pretty cold, right? Twelve-year-old boys lived life with a clear conscience in 1971. Also, Tara was nowhere as tough as Patty, so I wasn't all that worried.) Alyson was adorable, with long, brownish-blonde hair, a great smile and a great arm. I invited her to have a catch with us, which seemed like the easiest way to meet her, and it turned out that she threw and caught better than most of the guys I knew. She was a 12-year-old boy's dream — cute as hell and could play baseball. What more could you ask?

Upon returning to civilization, I was hastily made to remember who Ms. Keene was by none other than Tara herself. Incredibly, she failed to understand how I could be going out with her one minute, Alyson the next. "Well, you obviously haven't met Alyson," I informed her casually.

Enter Matty. He came along at precisely the right moment to take what had become a serious problem off my hands. Matty and Tara "went out" for just about three weeks before it was time for them to go their separate ways, which was par for the course at that age.

In Matty's mind, these events unfolded in a dramatically different manner. Whenever I introduce him to new people these days, and explain our history together, he inevitably informs them that he "stole Jimmy's girl Tara Keene away from him in sixth grade," saying it in such a way as to imply that I was soft and could do nothing about it. And he seems to believe this fantasy version of events. In the same breath he'll admit he has serious memory issues, instantly forgetting that he has just related a story from 40 years ago with unreserved conviction, as though it couldn't possibly have happened any other way.

I could go on and on but it would take hundreds of pages before I got to the CANCER part of the story. Suffice it to say that these four guys have been riding shotgun from the start. They are my go-to guys.

The good thing about having so many clever, sarcastic friends growing up was that everything you did had a competitive edge to it — you could either step up, or you could step aside. It kept us on our toes and really fine-tuned our social, psychological and physical dexterity, because getting left behind was not an option. For me, personally, it sent my developing willpower and ability to focus into overdrive, serving me well in many ways while getting me into a bit of trouble in others. With regard to the former, I can tell you beyond doubt that it was a primary factor in my cancer recovery. Yes, the surgery, the chemo, and my physiology (for which I can take no credit) were equally important, but without that willpower and intense focus I developed in Stuy Town back in the day, there's no way I could've pulled this off. No-sir-ree-Bob, this Beast had no idea who it was fucking with. It had never run into the likes of James P. Capuano, B.S.E. (Beast Slayer Extraordinaire).

Puhh!

Turkey on Whole Wheat, Dry

I started noticing something wasn't quite right around Christmas 2006. We were a week away from taking our first-ever winter family vacation. The kids had never even been on a plane before, and we were all pretty excited.

Meanwhile, I had been ignoring a dull ache in the lower right side of my abdomen for a while. It never really hurt that bad, and I knew, medically speaking, that if I continued to ignore it, it would just go away on its own. What's the worst it could be — appendicitis? An ulcer? No biggie. I'd deal with it when it became unbearable, my standard M.O.

In a momentary burst of good sense, I figured it wouldn't be such a good thing if we were in Punta Cana and my appendix exploded, so I acted like a big boy and actually called my doctor. Of course it was a Saturday, and he wasn't in.

"What is the purpose of your call, sir?" asked the woman at the service.

"He owes me quite a bit of money and I was wondering if I could stop by this afternoon to pick it up," I replied, after which I apologized and explained my quandary. "Any idea what it could be?" I asked her, like she would know.

Half an hour later, the doctor who was covering for

mine returned the call. He assured me it was probably nothing, and before long we were off to the Dominican Republic. Naturally, I saw no need to mention this little exchange to my wife, Dana, because that would have necessitated endless questions and scrutiny the entire trip. Far better to suffer silently than to have Dana stare and wait for me to spontaneously combust. And that's how she acted *before* I was diagnosed. You can imagine what it's like for me now that there's something legitimate for her to worry about.

No, all these petty things are better left unsaid — another of my time-honored M.O.'s.

Christmas, New Year's and Punta Cana came and went. We were back to the day-to-day slog of another bleak New York City winter.

By early summer the dull ache was a noticeable nuisance, one that was harder to ignore now that it was also making its presence known to others. No longer content to disrupt my day alone, it insisted on bringing innocent bystanders into the fray. And by innocent bystanders, I mean conference rooms full of colleagues at the giant financial information company where I was responsible for U.S. sales and account management, deli lines full of strangers, and all my unfortunate neighbors. The Beast likes to let everyone in on the fun. It doesn't discriminate on race, creed or color. In the eyes of the Beast, all tissue is created equal. It might have started out innocuously, but as soon as it realized I had zero control over its behavior, it grew bolder by the day. What began as a mild grumbling in my small intestine, much like a hunger pang, quickly grew to the decibels of the soundtrack to *Krakatoa, East of Java*. (For those of you not familiar with this movie from the late 1960s, it's about a gigantic island volcano in the Dutch East Indies that has the nerve to erupt and spoil an adulterous couple's efforts to salvage the dead husband's cargo ship full of priceless pearls.)

I'm not exaggerating. I'd be sitting in a meeting when my intestines would suddenly erupt, long and loud. Not only could I not conceal it, it was like a flashing neon arrow pointing directly to my abdomen. All eyes would fall upon me with that contemptuous "Jesus Christ, can't you at least run to the bathroom?" look. "Sorry about that, I'm having problems with my stomach," was my usual lame response.

As the eruptions began coming on fast and furious and I began doubling over in pain, it got tougher to dismiss these volcanic interludes. My colleagues grew concerned: "Dude — you'd better get to a doctor quick before you wreck all your suits," and "Holy shit — that's one of the scariest things I've ever heard. That came out of your body?"

You'd think my intestines wouldn't complain so loudly, since I ate less and less as the summer days dwindled away, to the point where my clothes fit me like they did that kid at the end of the movie *Big*. That's when people really began to notice.

"What?" I'd say dismissively. "Pencil thin is *in*."

By that point, I was working through all kinds of home remedies: milk of magnesia, Tums, Activea. My favorite was wintergreen Lifesavers. For a while there I was certain I had found the Holy Grail; I must have been popping them during some brief, dormant period in the eruption cycle, but I was convinced that my research had paid off.

I was virtually starving. Everything I tried to swallow, solid or liquid, was backing up into my small intestine and contributing to that terrifying noise. And, of course, momentarily crippling me.

I continued to keep this from Dana to the best of my ability. Fortunately, she was already out of the city for the summer with the kids. While she was aware I was having some "trouble," she was not aware of the extent to which my stomach was kicking my ass.

One lunchtime in my office with my friend Johnny Owen, I fessed up that I thought something might be seriously wrong.

"No shit," John observed in that sensitive way of his. Pointing to the uneaten sandwich on my desk, he turned up the dial. "Everyone's been telling you for two months to see a specialist," he said, "but you apparently think it makes more sense to experiment with turkey on whole wheat, because it's a well-known fact that a dry turkey sandwich has potent medicinal value."

"Are you done, jerk-off?" I shot back with equal sensitivity. "I'm simply eating very plain food until my stomach settles down."

While Johnny O. and his ilk were giving me shit for not doing enough to take care of my health, there was another equally vocal contingent abusing me for being a whiner.

I often drove my son Brandon, 12 at the time, and my daughter Julianna, 7, to school in the morning (which was completely ridiculous because it was only a six-block walk). Matty worked on 56th and Fifth and my office was in Times Square, so he would jump in the car too, and after I dropped off the kids we would take our time getting to work. It was kind of like those long lunch breaks I used to take with Tommy Dwyer, save for that we really did make it to work every day before nine.

We always took a different, circuitous route. Often, we'd find ourselves making the turn around the Duke Ellington memorial on the northeast end of Central Park before heading back down Fifth. Most people would kill for a 15-minute commute, and here we were, turning it into an hour-long cruise in New York City traffic each morning. "Wow, Madison Avenue is moving pretty nicely today," I'd say. "Whaddaya wanna do?"

"Cut over to Park," Matt might suggest. "The lights are all fucked up there and it usually creates a lot of traffic."

During these mid-summer rides, the eruptions flared up more frequently, much to my passenger's dismay. "Matty, I think there's something seriously wrong with me," I mentioned one morning.

"Stop being a little bitch," Matty shot back. "Just drive the fucking car".

In Matt's defense, John had been struggling with colorectal cancer for several years at that point, and another friend of ours, Miles, was in the middle of battling a variant of the Beast. Matty was unbelievably supportive of both of them. The thought of yet another close friend coming down with the "disease" was more than he could handle. (Looking back now, I think it's clear who was the bitch.)

My friend Roy was another story. He and I worked together for years. We'd become quite familiar with each others' strengths and weaknesses and exploited this knowledge as often as possible. Roy speaks with a very proper British accent, which he mistakenly believes makes everything he says sound interesting and intelligent. During our little smoking breaks in our "43rd Street, North" office, which was actually the back entrance to one of the theaters around the corner with a little overhang that protected us from the weather, Roy had zero tolerance for the merest mention of my health suspicions: "Oh, please," he'd say. "Is there no level to which you won't stoop for attention? Now you have *cancer*? Just move on with it then."

I was actually excited to inform him that they found a "mass" in my upper colon. We're very competitive with each other that way. When I mentioned to him that I was planning to write a memoir about my experience, he burst out laughing, which I took to mean: "Oh, so now you're a *writer*. Fantastic. Yet another feeble attempt at being noticed."

Well, what can Roy do? He's English.

A Disturbing Mass in My Cecum

Here's how I found out what I was in for: with Dana
and my Dad sitting in the emergency room one late
August morning at New York University Hospital in utter
panic while I lay comfortably on a gurney, happy as can be
from all the morphine, a young radiologist — he looked to
be about 14 — calmly informed me that there was "a
disturbing mass" in my "cecum," and it was completely
blocking my colon.

"Ahh," I thought to myself. "No wonder I'm in so
much pain, there's a disturbing mass in my cecum. Thank
God that's all it is."

Of course, I had no idea what or where my cecum
was, but it's amazing how wonderful everything sounds
given the right amount of morphine. The young doctor
went on to explain the location and purpose of one's
cecum, and what the disturbing mass might turn out to be,
and that's when I demanded more drugs — STAT.
(Wondering what STAT actually meant, I later took the
time to look it up. Turns out it's both an acronym, "Sooner
Than Already There," AND an abbreviation of the Latin
"statim," which means "immediately".) The physician in
charge told me I'd need to be admitted to surgery
immediately, no time to waste. (I guess he wasn't familiar
with "STAT.") In a very loving, morphine-induced mood, I

thanked the doctor, whose name I cannot recall, for being such a good friend. "Let's do it!" I said thickly. (My tongue felt like one of those giant Amazon leeches and I was having trouble convincing my words to scramble around it).

Luckily for me, Dana was there to take charge. She explained to the staff that unless I had only a few hours left to live, there was no way I would be admitted until we had cleared this with our good friend Dr. Zvi Fuks, a world-renowned oncologist at Memorial Sloan-Kettering Cancer Center.

After much haggling and my signature, which I don't remember giving, on a release form, I followed Dana out onto First Avenue at 5 a.m. as we trudged home to make that call.

*

Genetically speaking, that moment when I followed Dana out of the hospital like a good little doggie was an anomaly because it had never been written into my cultural DNA to behave that way. Nowhere in that code are instructions for me to blindly do whatever it is my wife says I should do. Within the culture that was handed down to me, it was evident at all times that the man called the shots and the woman did what the man said. Rationally, of course, I can't justify that, but I grew up in a big Italian family where it was just expected.

My mother's parents were from Sicily, and my father's from Bari and Naples. Jeez, talk about stubborn and demanding. Sunday dinners — that incredibly auspicious consequence of my heritage for anyone who enjoys food — were alternately played out at each grandparents' apartment and included literally everyone in the family, as well as certain hangers-on: mothers, fathers, brothers, sisters, cousins, aunts and uncles, in-laws, Sal the Butcher (whose wife was too sick to cook), and so on. These were relatively small city apartments, so there was never enough room for everyone at the table. Yet, magically, my grandparents always managed to make it work. We laughed, we ate, we joked, we argued and cried. Then we laughed and ate some more. Dinner always consisted of several pounds of pasta, three different kinds of meat, a minimum of two vegetables, plus salad, bread and vino, and the whole affair typically took not less than three hours to complete. The meal was considered *finito* only when the last of the espresso / sambuca / anisette was gone, and the fruit, nuts, and "pizza dolce" were cleared from the table.

That's when the men would typically retire to the living room to smoke and watch television while the women, from the oldest to the youngest, cleaned up and put everything away. It wasn't because the men in my family were mean or lazy, but because that's the way it had been done in the Old Country for generations. It was normal for them to behave that way, and the women bought into it too.

Those were the days, my friend. It's virtually impossible to get away with that particular brand of chauvinism in the 21st Century, regardless of what culture you happen to be descended from.

Did You Mean: *"disturbing mass, cecum, cancer, prognosis, survival rate, adenocarcinoma ..."?*

Boy, the next time some doctor tells me NOT to go on the Internet to research some medical condition because I'm not trained to decipher that sort of information, goddammit, I'm gonna listen to him.

Dr. Fuks told me loud and clear over the phone that the one thing Dana and I absolutely could not do was surf the Web for a diagnosis. "Jimmy, listen to me — you and Dana are not trained to comprehend the volumes of information you will come across on the Internet," he warned. "Promise me you won't start snooping around. We won't know ourselves what the diagnosis is until the gastroenterologist goes in and gets a stain. Do you understand that?"

"I do, Zvi," I said. "A stain, yes. Well, thank you for giving me the heads-up."

"Don't be silly," he said. "You will listen to me and I will arrange for everything you need. Your surgeon, your oncologist. Dr. Shike will do a colonoscopy as soon as possible to determine what it is we're dealing with here."

"That's fantastic, Zvi," I said. "Thank you so much. You can count on me to do whatever I need to do. I know

I'm in great hands."

The first thing Dana and I did the second we hung up the phone was to grab our laptops and start furiously Googling all kinds of shit we had heard, as well as shit we thought we had heard. We typed in words and phrases like: "disturbing mass, cecum, cancer, prognosis, colon, survival rate." And got back results like: "Surgical planes were created to resect the colonic mass en bloc with the invaded appendix, ascending / transverse colon, loop of ileum, and right abdominal wall / retroperitoneum. Liver, ileocolic mesentery, and para-aortic regions......"

Just as Zvi had promised, the results were completely and horribly overwhelming, and neither of us had the slightest idea what any of it meant.

But I've always sucked at taking orders. When I was a teen, I used to go head to head with my father all the time because I innately hate being told what to do. Whether it's something as small as throwing out the garbage or as big as saving the planet from vampire zombie dogs because I know the secret death incantation, it makes no difference. If someone tells me to do it, it's an automatic argument. My poor mother hated those scenes. She would always make those big, fluffy eyes at me behind my father's back, as if to say, "Why can't you just shut up for once in your life?"

I find it equally disturbing to be told I can't do something. The family joke, which my father still throws up at me to this day, is my alleged rant of "it's not fair!"

whenever I don't like or agree with something, but I honestly don't see what's funny about that. (Oh, I'm sorry — was I supposed to wear those ridiculous Skips when all my friends had high white Chuck Taylor All Stars? I'd rather go barefoot.)

My mom could never bring herself to be the heavy, and she was extraordinarily tolerant. My brother and I, along with our cousin Joseph — who was more like a third son than a nephew — used to drive her crazy, constantly ignoring her pleas to stop propping the coffee table up on one end to use as a slide, and to not fill our air rifles with dirt from the plant and milk from the refrigerator to shoot out of our third-floor window. It drove her crazy when we sat on the turntable, which was housed in a big furniture console, and took turns spinning around, pushing each other as fast as we could (my parents eventually put a special lock on the console but it didn't take long for us to figure out a way around it).

My two younger sisters instinctively understood that if they just did the opposite of whatever it was we were doing, they wouldn't get into any trouble. Laura, born four years after me, would cry at the drop of a hat, so she was given a wide berth anyway. Rosanne, born five years after Laura, was the baby of the family and far too cute to get mad at regardless of what she did, so she never had anything to worry about.

The rest of us took full advantage of Mom's uncommonly kind nature and would push things until she would eventually bite her wrists in frustration.

In baseball, a third-base coach uses signs to tell the batter and the runners what to do. There are hundreds of signs, but none of them matter until the coach gives the "indicator" sign, which could be touching the brim of his hat, touching his belt — anything really, as long as the players know the indicator ahead of time. The very next sign after that is the "hot" sign, the one that matters. Biting her wrist was my mother's indicator, followed by a fist in the air — the "hot" sign, signaling that her head was about to explode. That's when we knew it was time to back off.

More often than not, my father would be alerted to our shenanigans by the teeth marks on my mom's wrists and we'd be in for it. But trouble was never a physical concern in my family. My dad never raised a hand to any of us. He didn't have to. He was a New York City police sergeant, and the "angry cop" look he threw our way was scary enough. I've had the pleasure of watching him in action many times over the years as he battled crime while he was off-duty. One Saturday night, while on his way home from a Knights of Columbus dance with my mother, he scared off a mugger. It was about 3 a.m. and he and my mom were in fine shape (they always knew how to have a good time) when Sgt. Pasquale Capuano's spidey sense picked up on a guy who was trailing a little too close behind them. Before the guy could make his move, Dad told Mom to pretend she twisted her ankle (she always enjoyed playing a supporting role in these little cop dramas) so he could bend down and pull his snub-nosed .38 revolver from his ankle holster.

"Whoa, man!" said the hood to the sergeant. "Whatchu doin' wit dat gun? I ain't doin' nuttin' to you."

"You're goddamn right you're not, you sonofabitch," said the sergeant to the hood. "I don't wanna hear you talk, I just wanna see you run down that block. Move now before I make it so you can't move at all!"

Needless to say, the guy took off. About halfway down the block, the perp slowed down to scope out an elderly couple also on their way home from the dance. "I can still put six in you from here" my father yelled, loud and clear.

When he was first starting out on "the job" Dad's spidey sense wasn't quite so fine-tuned. While walking the beat one day in Murray Hill as a young cop, he noticed a moving van parked in front of a building on East 36th Street (right next door to the building Dana grew up in, coincidentally). Two or three young guys appeared to be having trouble getting some large pieces of furniture out the front door. Nice guy that my dad was, he walked over to lend a hand:

"You guys look like you could use a little help," said Officer Capuano.

"That would be great, Officer," one of the movers said. "Some of these pieces are mighty heavy and we need to get this job done before evening."

"It's great to have a job like this where I get to help people every day," the young patrolman thought, feeling very self-righteous. My father spent the next two hours helping those gentlemen complete the difficult task of entirely emptying the ground-floor apartment of a well-dressed, middle-aged woman, who later reported the burglary.

While Dad never had to go quite so far as to pull a gun on us to make us stop doing whatever it was we shouldn't have been doing, he did throw a hammer "toward" me once in utter frustration.

"Goddammit, if I see you sweep one more piece of chicken into that hole I'm gonna lose my friggin' mind," he articulated yet again, just in case I missed it the first four times. "I told you to pick it up and throw it in the bin."

"Alright, alright! God, what is the big deal?" I answered, defiantly.

I mean, so what if I was sweeping rotten pieces of chicken into a hole leading to the basement of the shuttered Kentucky Fried Chicken storefront where we were selling Christmas trees that year? And so what if that basement happened to be where Dad was storing those trees each night? Jeez, he makes such a big deal out of everything.

When I got back to the repulsive task he had burdened me with, I saw there was only one lousy little piece of months-old chicken left to dispose of. "Shit," I thought to myself. "What harm could there be in sweeping one more piece of chicken into that hole, considering that I've already swept in about 50 pieces? " As I boldly nudged the chicken toward the rim with my broom, I looked up in time to see the hammer my father had been using to build some God-awful Christmas-tree-holding structure come flying toward me, passing uncomfortably close to my head.

"Jesus Christ! I can't believe you just threw a hammer at my head!" I said, not very bravely. "Why would you wanna hit me with a hammer?"

"If I wanted to hit you with a hammer, the hammer would have hit you," he said. "Go ahead — sweep that last piece of chicken into that hole and see what happens."

I always knew when I could get away with calling his bluff, but this was not one of those times. Being somewhat obsessive-compulsive when it comes to straight lines and completing tasks in a unified manner, I'm still freaked out to this day that I couldn't sweep that last piece of fucking chicken into that hole so I could put a mental checkmark on a task properly completed.

For the most part though, discipline consisted of "stay in your room for the next month," or, "you're not to eat another thing until tomorrow morning." But these were not idle threats. If Dad said it, he meant it. The latter was easy, as my brother and I knew that at some point my mom would sneak us a pack of Yodels or some equally healthy taste treat. There was no way she was gonna let her boys go to bed hungry.

Which reminds me, when I was little I used to actually call my brother "Brother," as though that were his name. I did that not because it was '60s hipster slang, as in "What's up, my brother?" I did it because he made me, from the moment I could speak. I guess it was cute when I was 2 or 3, but it sounded a little strange coming out of the mouth of a 10-year-old, especially in front of my friends. We used to share a room and he would often leverage the still of the night to inform me that if I ever dared to call him by his real name, not only would he never speak to me again, he'd have me sent back to my real family in Africa as well. He's only a year and a half older, but he was a master manipulator and would convince me to do all kinds of crazy shit — it was his idea to spin on the turntable and shoot milk-dirt at people, not mine. I think he's still pissed that I don't call him "Brother" anymore. His name is Richard and I used to make my sons call him "Uncle Dick" in front of visitors. What goes around, as they say.

My father would always try to use reason when disciplining us, but it was a waste of time with me because I wasn't the least bit reasonable. When he'd finally give up and tell me to sit on my bed for three days and not move, I'd say, "Fine, I'll sit on my bed for *five* days and not move," and I'd do it just to win my point. I wasn't going to be the one to cave. This stubbornness is an inherited characteristic that would come in handy when battling the Beast.

*

Everyone loved my mother. She had that rare gift of making you feel like the most important person in the world, even if she had just met you. (My father-in-law, Jerry, was like that too. Either I was incredibly lucky to have two people like that in my immediate family, or it just proves that I *am* the most important person in the world. Either way, it was always a pleasure to be around the two of them.)

Sadly, my mom passed away while I was writing this book. She suffered for years with emphysema, the result of three packs of cigarettes a day for a good portion of her life. She essentially suffocated, very slowly, over the course of 10 years. What a horrible disease. But she never lost sight of the humor or the absurdity in everything, and she never stopped laughing, right up until the end.

Like my dad, Mom spent her entire life in New York, always within a three-block radius of where she grew up. The two of them met while attending the Epiphany School: a young Pasquale James Capuano and Ann Marie Burgio. Her mom and dad owned a grocery store on 20th Street and Third Avenue called "Victory Market," named for the good guys winning the Second World War, and all of the television and movie stars who lived in Gramercy Park at the time shopped there. There was no such thing as a "supermarket" back then — Victory Market was all they had — and my grandparents were on a first-name basis with each and every one of them. My brother and I used to call my grandfather Papa, so they called him "Papa Tony."

James Cagney, Tina Louise ("Ginger" on *Gilligan's Island*), and the Oscar-nominated actress Brenda Vaccaro — an eclectic list — all restocked their refrigerators with Papa Tony's produce. (When Brenda was just starting out, Papa Tony gave her groceries and some cash from time to time to help her make ends meet.)

But for me, being so young, there was only one actress who made an impression on me, and a lasting impression it was.

The Wizard of Oz was (and quite possibly still is) the scariest movie of all time. Every kid who's ever seen it has had recurring nightmares about flying monkeys carrying them off to the lair of the Wicked Witch.

That dream was nothing compared to what I had to contend with in real life. Imagine standing around your grandfather's store, lazily spraying the vegetables (as well as the odd customer or two) with cold water to keep them fresh, only to look up and find your worst nightmare materializing in front of your eyes: Margaret Hamilton, the actual fucking Wicked Witch of the West, walking into the store with her arms out, looking to scoop up little Jimmy in a great, big witch hug. Holy shit! There was nothing more terrifying than that.

"Here Jimmy, come give Margaret a hug!" she'd insist.

"Who the fuck is Margaret?" I'd ask myself. "She's not fooling me." And Dorothy should've known better, too. I would drop the hose and run full speed across the store and into the waiting arms of my mother.

I can't think of anything more comforting than having her be there to save me, each and every time. Boy, it doesn't seem to matter whether you're five, twenty-five, or fifty; when your mom goes, a big part of you goes with her. It makes you feel like you've been left alone, regardless of who's by your side, and it creates a void that I'm willing to bet can never be filled. It makes you realize how vulnerable and childlike you really are. And every now and then, when there's no one else around and the witches and the flying monkeys are doing their best to scoop you up, you catch yourself thinking: "I want my mommy."

Fucking emphysema. Puhh!

A Terrace!
You Think I Can Smoke a Cigar Out There?

While taking a stroll around the 15th floor at MSK-CC with Dana one afternoon prior to my surgery, checking out my new digs, we noticed a beautiful little terrace outside the family room with picnic tables, lounge chairs and the like, and I got very excited. The sun was shining, it was a beautiful early fall day, and the terrace was pretty much empty, so we decided to step out. It was fantastic.

"They really do everything they can to make you feel comfortable around here," I said.

"Yes, this is really nice," said Dana. "At least you'll be able to get some fresh air and not feel so much like you're in a hospital."

"Yup. I'm psyched," said I. "You think I can smoke a cigar out here?"

Dana, killjoy that she was, thought that would pretty much be frowned upon in those parts.

"Why?" I insisted. "What's the big deal? I can sit in that corner over there and smoke and not bother anyone. I'm gonna call Matt and have him bring up a couple of stogies."

"Yeah, well, just to remind you; this is a CANCER HOSPITAL, moron," said my sweet, pretty wife. "I can pretty much guarantee they won't let you sit out there and smoke a cigar."

"That's such bullshit," was all I could say. But "it's not fair" was what I was thinking.

I've always had an obsession with cigars. Nothing Freudian, mind you. Even Freud is rumored to have said "sometimes a cigar is just a cigar" when questioned about his fondness for sticking burning-hot cylinders into his mouth. (How convenient of Freud to exempt himself from being subject to his own psycho-babble). From an early age I can remember my father and his friends smoking cigars on vacation at the Police Camp. (You're probably about to conjure up an image of all of us dressed in little cop uniforms, walking around cuffing each other and handing out tickets, but the "Police Camp" was actually a beautiful resort in the Catskills owned by the NYC Police Department. It provided an affordable break from city life for cops and their families. Its formal name was the Police Recreation Centre, but all of us wily veterans referred to it simply as "the Camp." All my best memories from childhood come from the family vacations we took there. In fact, that's where I met Alyson Bruu, whose dad was also a cop). There was something about the social aspect of smoking and talking and laughing that has always intrigued me. Whenever I light up a cigar today I can feel and smell those vacations from 40 years ago.

I first started experimenting with cigars in my late teens. John and I would split a pack of Tiparillo's, those cheap little stogies with the cigar holders built into them, and we'd sit around smoking and pretending we actually enjoyed it. He wasn't really into it but I convinced him it was something we needed to do. Most of the time, we'd just laugh about how ridiculous we looked.

John used to deliver something or other after school, I can't remember what, on a motorized Moped scooter, and I have a very clear memory of him pulling up to me one day wearing that giant helmet that made him look like the Great Gazoo from the Flintstones cartoon, and a Tiparillo sticking out of the corner of his mouth, and I started crying I was laughing so hard. John just flicked the cigar at me and drove off to make his delivery. It was at that point, at the height of ridiculousness, that I realized if I were going to keep on smoking cigars, I'd have to get more serious about it.

"I'm out," John informed me. "These things suck. And don't even pretend you enjoy smoking them."

"Whatever," I replied. "You're a shitty cigar smoker anyway."

Matty, however, was more than happy to join in when I went slightly more upscale to Macanudos. He and I have been smoking cigars together ever since.

In spite of Dana's unwavering assertion that I would NOT be able to smoke on the Sloan Kettering terrace, I called Matty and asked him to bring up a couple of Davidoff robustos, which make for a quick, satisfying smoke, to which he replied, "You're in a CANCER HOSPITAL, jerk-off. They're not gonna let us smoke a cigar out there."

"That's such bullshit," was all I could say.

I Know, But I'm Not Allowed to Tell You

Dana and I had been together for roughly 24 years by September of 2007, inclusive of nearly five years' worth of scattered breakups and reunions before we got married in 1988. The way that worked was that I would break up with her, she would start seeing someone else, I would get pissed, make her miserable, win her back, swear my undying love, and then repeat the cycle a bit down the road. She would agree with most of what I just said, except for the word "pissed." She'd probably use the word "jealous," but she'd be wrong. I'm not the jealous type — I just don't like it when other guys start messin' around with my ex-girlfriend.

We met in college. Our school was the State University of New York / College at New Paltz, in the foothills of the Shawangunk and Catskill Mountains. (New Paltz was an "artsy," hippie college in the '60s and '70s, and I went there mainly to grow my hair, live in the country, and study music from every angle. The place also had a reputation as a serious party school, but I don't remember any of that.) Dana was a senior and I was finishing up year two of a two-month post-graduation extension during which I pursued my rock and roll dreams with my partner Gary Fitzgerald. I began playing music when I was 8 or 9 and knew then that the only thing I wanted to be if I ever grew up was a successful recording artist. By the time we graduated, Gary and I firmly believed we were just about as good as Lennon & McCartney at penning hits, and that a record deal (followed by much fame and fortune) was imminent, although we were already a little late, based on the time-line we had established for ourselves.

During that two-year period, Gary and I earned our living playing music three or four nights a week. This included six months out west, where we presented ourselves as an acoustic guitar duo to ski resorts and bars because that was so much easier than carting a whole band around. It was also far more lucrative, as it meant splitting the cash two ways rather than several. We both swear MTV got the whole "Unplugged" idea after seeing us play one night. It was an amazing time.

I made the mistake once of telling a friend about it within earshot of my son Danny, who listened as I punctuated the story with, "Yup, the best two years of my life." "Really?" Danny said. "*Those* were the best two years of your life? I guess having kids and stuff didn't make that big an impression then."

"Not what I meant, Danny. Not what I meant." What else could I say? But it kinda *was* what I meant. It was a ridiculously good time.

Gary and I became acquainted with each other inadvertently during sophomore year when we signed up for the same piano class, a prerequisite for a Music Theory and Composition degree and not a throwaway class for someone who already knew how to play the piano. Fencing and swimming were throwaway classes for someone who already knew how to play the piano and was seeking an undergraduate degree in music theory and composition.

We had this nutty professor, a sweetheart of a guy named Dr. Landau, who was roughly 117 years old. He was explaining tonality and how sound is created during our first class of the semester when he abruptly stuck his head inside the piano and began singing, "GEEEEEEE, GEEEEEEE, GEEEEEE," over and over in his 117-year-old voice to show us that he could make the G string inside the piano vibrate and come alive simply by producing a sound that vibrated at the same frequency. Gary and I had a good deal of success utilizing this technique on women in 1978, despite the fact that G strings were not yet fashionable.

While hysterical on its own, what made it even funnier was that the professor repeated this exercise with his head inside the piano for two solid minutes before he finally got it right. No one in the class wanted to hurt his feelings, but there was no way we could contain ourselves. When he finally came up for air his glasses were crooked, his tie was twisted up, and what was left of his hair was pointing in six different directions. He then proceeded to explain what was going to be on the quiz the following week, but I didn't catch any of it because I was still laughing.

"What did he just say?" I asked the guy next to me.

"Look, if you think I'm gonna sit here and take notes for you while you fuck around for an hour and a half, you're outta your fucking mind," said the guy. "Start paying some attention and leave me the fuck alone."

"That's pretty funny," I told him. "What's your name, douche-bag?"

His name was Gary, and we've been friends and collaborators ever since.

Gary happened to have his acoustic guitar with him that fateful day. "Mind if I check it out?" I asked. "I've never played an Ovation before."

"You know how to play?" Gary said, sarcastically.

"No, I was thinking I could learn right here on the spot," I replied. "How hard could it be?" Then I played and sang, much to Gary's delight: *Dear Prudence, won't you come out to play-ay-ay / Dear Prudence, greet the brand new day-ay-ay aye…*"

"Nice," said Gary. "You can play and sing. And you're a Beatles fan. Feel like getting together later and playing a bit?"

"You know how to play?" I responded. "Just messin'. I'm definitely into it. Where do you live?"

"Riverside Apartments, on Huguenot Street — right near the Old Stone Houses."

"GET THE FUCK OUTTA HERE!!" I said. That's where I was living too.

We got together later that day and worked up a version of *Dear Prudence* that was to become our signature opening song. The rest, as they say, is an unsung footnote in music history, but Gary remains one of the most talented, funny and sarcastic bastards I've ever met.

Upon returning to New York, I spent eight years in a low-level job within Citibank's Latin American Debt Restructuring Group (and by "low-level" I mean "low-paying") while still aggressively pursuing a career in music with Gary and a core group of musician friends. With my degree in music theory and composition, Latin American debt restructuring seemed like an obvious next step. I'd work all day and gig at night. It was easy enough when we were playing in the city, but there were plenty of times when I'd get a call at 2 p.m. from my buddy Peter (a fantastic musician who earned the nickname "the Most," because he is), telling me we had a gig in Poughkeepsie at eight. Or in Kingston, or Woodstock. I'd rush home, pack up my equipment, drive upstate, and get to the venue with three minutes to set up and be ready to play. At the end of the night, I had to break down my equipment, re-pack the car, drive back home, unpack, and hope to get an hour or two of sleep before restructuring some more debt for Argentina, Venezuela and Brazil. On a stellar night, I'd walk out of the gig with twenty bucks in my pocket. All very glamorous. Needless to say, my parents were less than delighted with my career decisions and general judgment from 1981 through roughly 1991.

My son Nick was born in 1989. Danny came along in 1992, followed by Brandon in 1995. After a bit of a breather, Julianna was born in 2000 and our family was complete. We were six people, big and small, living in a three-bedroom, one-bath apartment in Stuy Town. Having grown up there, I guess I never really noticed how cramped we were.

If I had to use a single word to describe each of my children, and speculate as to what their future selves are likely to be doing, I suppose the word for Nick would be "cautious." He doesn't like to leave himself exposed. His natural inclination is to evaluate a situation, leave no stone unturned, and position himself for success (which he generally achieves). However, if for some reason he's not satisfied with the result, it's not uncommon for him to slip back into a more childlike version of himself, which is an amazing transformation. But the older he gets, the less we see of "little Nicky." He's extremely pragmatic and will always do the right thing. He definitely enjoys the finer things in life, which he's happy to work hard to obtain. A financial services professional through and through.

For Danny, I would use the word "clever." He's very quick-witted and humorous in his observations, and has an uncanny ability to remember facts, quotes and sports statistics. I can never tell if he actually knows all these facts and stats he throws out there or if he's just making shit up, but it doesn't matter; he says things with such conviction that you'd never think to challenge him. He's passionate and therefore quick-tempered, but his kind heart always leads him back home. The ideal job for him would be a sportscaster or some type of TV personality. I'd tune in to watch even if he weren't my son.

Brandon is free-spirited. He has no bid for structure and, like someone else we know, hates being told what to do. He can accomplish just about anything he puts his mind to, but he's very selective. While Nicky is an excellent singer / songwriter in his own right, and considers it a hobby, Brandon is the scion who will most likely follow in my footsteps with regard to pursuing a calling. It could be music, which he takes to naturally, or it could be teaching — he's very kind, and great with little kids. He's also a fucking nut-job, but I mean that in the best possible way.

Julianna — well, what can a man say about his only daughter, who just happens to be the baby of the family? That she's beautiful, smart, talented and sweet? None of those words would be strong enough or meaningful enough to encapsulate her. I guess I could say she's kind-hearted and loyal and would never purposely hurt someone's feelings or blindly follow the crowd, but that wouldn't do her justice either. As far as occupation goes, she definitely inherited the entertainment gene and loves an audience. I could easily see her being a successful actress one day. It's almost impossible to come up with one single word to describe her, but since I've put myself in this position I guess I would have to say that her

50

nickname, "Jules," would be a good place to start — she is indeed a jewel.

*

In September 2007, after decades of being a large family stuffed into a small space, I suddenly had my own room for the first time since 1988. I was in Sloan Kettering prior to my first surgery, and my "roommate," Bill, had just been discharged. He was back home with his wife, Sarah, and son, Cliff, recuperating from his second surgery (his cancer was back for a return engagement after a couple of years on the road). This left me on my own for several days.

Bill was the editor-in-chief of a quintessential music industry publication called *Modern Drummer Magazine*. He was also an accomplished jazz drummer and an all around gem of a human being. We bunked together for about two weeks before he was discharged. Within a couple of hours we were acting as if we'd known each other since the first grade. We figured our souls must have been acquainted in past lives; how else to explain such an instant connection (other than that we were both musicians stuck in a hospital room together with similar, horrendous health issues)? We kept in touch regularly via email and phone after he went home, planning steak dinners and picking out concerts we'd attend together the following fall once our treatments had ended .

"I can get us backstage at just about any show," Bill mentioned.

"I'm in," I mentioned right back.

Months later, he informed me that a new spot had shown up in a recent scan. "It's small, no big deal," he said. "I'm not all that worried about it, pally." (Bill affectionately referred to his friends as "pally.") He said he was about to start on an experimental drug that had shown great promise.

"Well, what's it called?" I said. "What are the stats on the control studies? What's the unique component of this treatment that makes it more viable than the others and what kind of side effects are we talking about here?" We had both become unwitting experts in cancer care by then.

I started to get concerned when his normally lengthy emails were down to one or two lines, with too much time elapsing between missives. I was sitting in my office one day when my cell phone rang and Bill's name popped up on the screen. "Finally," I said into the mouthpiece of my Blackberry. "Where the hell have you been, Willie?" But it wasn't Bill's voice that answered; it was Sarah's. I could feel my stomach tie itself into a knot. She didn't have to say it; I knew the instant I heard her voice.

"Things really got worse for him right after Thanksgiving," she told me. "He became more and more incoherent, and was having a difficult time even holding a conversation. Thankfully, he got to be with his family for the holiday."

"Wow, Sarah," I said. "I have some emails from him dated right around that time. I knew because of how brief they were, just a couple of sentences each, that something wasn't right, but he never let on that things were that bad. I would have come out to see him if I had known."

"I'm really surprised he was able to respond to emails," Sarah said. "He was so out of it at that point. That's amazing."

Bill's passing hit me hard. I closed my office door after I hung up and cried like a baby. A few short weeks before, I had lost a friend at work — another victim of the ugly fucking Beast. I felt like I was having a nervous breakdown. Not only was I crushed by the realization that my friends were dying, I was being forced to face the reality of my situation as well, which at that point wasn't overflowing with promise. (Hope was readily available; promise was behaving like a selfish motherfucker). It wasn't until weeks later that I was able to pull myself together. It was after re-reading one of Bill's emails, in which he reported that after many grueling rounds of treatment that seemed to be destroying the one small tumor they were targeting, several other small spots had appeared nearby. Ever the optimist, he signed off with, "Well pally, not all good, but not horrible either. Just have to keep fighting."

Here was a guy who had just been told, in boxing

parlance, that the Beast was pounding him mercilessly in his own corner with left hooks and right uppercuts to the head and there were still two and a half minutes left in the round (the equivalent of forever to a boxer that's hurt). "Oh well," he figured, "just have to keep fighting."

I've been carrying his words around with me for three years now. One day, when our souls reconnect, I'm gonna let Bill know just how much they've meant to me.

*

At first, Dana and I did everything we could to keep our son Nick from finding out about my little predicament. Other than a week here and a week there, he had never been away on his own, and he had just started freshman year at Hamilton College. But smart kids are not to be fooled. He called my cell phone one evening while I was lying in my hospital bed in my "private" room, a day or two before my surgery, and I tried to play it cool — very difficult when you're stoned from all those meds.

"Hey, no problem here," I assured him. "No reason for concern."

"That's such bullshit," he said. I don't know where he got language like that. "I'm dropping out for the semester and coming home."

"You are NOT coming home," I responded, which

was pretty authoritative considering all those mellow-making drugs I was on. "If you really want to help me, stay in school and do the best you can. I'll be fine. How did you figure out what was going on, anyway?"

"I called the house and Jules answered," Nick said. "When I asked why I could hear Mimi [my mother-in-law, Diane] in the background, Jules said she's sleeping there. When I asked why, she said, 'I know, but I'm not allowed to tell you'."

I'm gonna have to cut Jules some slack on that one. After all, she was only seven at the time, and I'd been up at Sloan-Kettering for a couple of weeks at that point. If the same situation arose today, I have no doubt whatsoever that she would handle the call like a pro, lying with complete an utter conviction. That's my girl.

And How Long Will You Be
Staying With Us, Sir?

Thirty days.

That's a long time, thirty days.

Staying anywhere that's not your home for thirty days is generally intolerable. You can't get comfortable, it's not your own bed, the food sucks, and you can't walk around naked. Thirty days in a hospital is the equivalent of ninety days just about anywhere else you don't want to be. Except for prison. Maybe.

I had no idea when I was admitted that I'd be there that long. Because of that pesky little eating and drinking disorder I had, it seems that the Beast was able to persuade some neighboring organs to get in on the action. The reason I felt like I was knocking on death's door by the time I got to the hospital was because I was knocking on death's door.

It wasn't the Beast itself that was bringing me down, it was its effect on the rest of my system. My inability to swallow requisite amounts of food and drink (including scotch) for several weeks had left me on the verge of double kidney failure. I was so dehydrated it took over two weeks to get the fluid level in my body normalized enough for Dr. Helm to work his magic in the operating room, exorcising the Beast from my tender little abdomen with chanting and sharp knives. That's how pissed off my kidneys were. Good thing the morphine pump and I were on excellent terms by then. It's funny, I've always thought of the kidneys as second-class organs in the abdominal-chest hierarchy of the body. The heart, lungs and liver were the big men on campus. Yes, the small intestine and the colon tend to receive significant attention, and the stomach and pancreas get honorable mention from time to time, but I have to tell you I have new-found respect for the kidneys. Just because you can technically survive on one doesn't diminish their value. If you don't believe me, just let your body dry out for a week or two and then tell me if I'm lying. No sir; I say the kidneys have got it going on. My hat's off to them.

So how did they rehydrate me and provide me with enough nutrition to sustain life as we know it if I wasn't able to eat or drink? I had lost my appetite weeks before, and had given up on trying to force food down my throat because every time I did, I'd get smacked down by debilitating pain. Fuck it, I figured; it's not worth the trouble anymore. I was on the verge of giving up altogether. And then one afternoon these two lovely Asian women entered my room dressed in scrubs, carrying surgical utensils, and dragging some kind of monitoring device behind them.

"Good afternoon, ladies, how can I help you?" I asked in that happy-go-lucky morphine-addled kind of way.

"We are here to help *you*," one of them corrected me. "We are going to insert a PICC line into your body so that we can feed you intravenously."

"Hmm," I said. "Insert a PICC line into my body and feed me intravenously? Somehow I don't think I'm going to like that. Do we need to go into an operating room for this?"

"No, no, no. We will do the procedure right here in your room. Everything is sterile and it will only take ten minutes. Don't worry, this is a very simple procedure and we have done it many times before."

"Is it going to hurt?" I bravely inquired.

"No, no, no; you won't even feel it. We are going to insert the line through a vein under your right bicep and snake it through your chest cavity into the main aorta going into your heart."

"Whoa, wait a second please," I said quite cordially. "That sounds horribly wrong in so many ways. Do the doctors know you're doing this?"

"Of course, silly," the nurse I no longer cared for replied. "The doctors ordered it."

Still not convinced, I asked about the anesthesia. "No, no, no; no anesthesia," they assured me. "It will not hurt. You will feel a little pinch when we make the incision and that is all."

"You're making an incision and you're not gonna give

Science Made Simple:
Lesson 1 — Good Cells / Bad Cells

When one thinks of cancer, one understandably thinks of expressions like "killer," "vicious" and "doomed." Now that I've come face to face with the Beast, I look at it a little differently.

In my current view, the Beast in and of itself is not very tough at all. More like a bully, really. It's basically a bunch of freakishly abnormal cells that have figured out how to reproduce freakish little replicas of themselves until they get big enough to strong-arm the well-intentioned cells in our body — those cells that quietly go about their business in our organs, lymph nodes, connective tissue and so forth, not bothering anyone. These freak-cells travel around the bloodstream until they find a group of normal cells cowering in the corner because there aren't enough antibodies around at that moment to stick up for them (probably off smacking cold and flu bugs around somewhere). These clever little bastards work their way in by pretending to be friendly and cool, and before you know it they've taken over. With time, they grow bigger and uglier and start turning on their host — which constitutes very poor manners in the extreme. Major organs that used to get along beautifully, peacefully co-existing and doing their own thing, turn against one another.

If this goes on unnoticed for too long, well, that's when things start to get really unpleasant. The liver can't live anymore, the kidneys can't kid, the intestines can't intest. Once it gets to that point, it's time to call in "the pros from Dover," as my friend Bill Cassato would say.

Bill and I worked together for many years. About 10 years ago, we traveled on an urgent trip to a very important customer in Newport Beach, California, who was on the verge of becoming a former customer (yet another rough assignment for the boys). It was a delicate situation, but we handled it beautifully. As we were walking out of the building and into a picture-perfect, blue-sky California day, I figured I'd call the office to report our successful outcome. Bill grabbed the cell phone from my hand.

"Jimmy, Jimmy, Jimmy," he intoned. "*Never* report good news that fast. Far better to let them wonder, imagining the brutal negotiation we had to go through before we finally pulled this puppy back from the brink. Bad news you report immediately; good news you milk for all it's worth."

We ended up having dinner that night near the hotel we were staying at in Newport Beach, and soon took over the club. As I sang with the band and Bill danced with some of the more "mature" women who had gathered on the dance floor to take part in the festivities, one of them turned to him and asked, "Who are you guys, anyway?" To which he replied, "Why, we're the pros from Dover,

Ma'am." It was an expression used in the 1970 movie *M*A*S*H** to describe consultants that are brought in to troubleshoot difficult situations, and Cassato's timing that night was brilliant. We've been using the phrase ever since.

*

Okay, what was it I was saying about good cells and bad cells? Oh, yeah, I remember now:

Puhh! Ugly little mutant replicant freaks. You think you're so bad? Puhh! Say hello to my little friends Dr. Keltner and Dr. Helm. While you're at it, meet their associates: Avastin, Oxaliplatin and Flourouracil. Not so tough *now*, are you, you motherfuckers?

I pause here to remind you that once you are in the club you can say whatever you damn well please about the Beast. And you can curse without being offensive, which is nice.

But Let's Get Back to the Thirty Days ...

Time in a hospital is *hard* time. There are no time outs, no whistles to stop the play. You would think "sleeping" constitutes a time out, but it doesn't. How about lying in your bed two hours after surgery? Nope. Maybe going to the bathroom would warrant a whistle? Sorry.

In a hospital, time as we know it doesn't exist. Every moment swishes into the next in a sort of free-form, multi-directional manner. Past, present and future are indistinguishable. It's Einstein's Theory of Relativity in its most practical form.

If you are somehow able to ignore all the gauges and thermometers and close your eyes for some shuteye, you're still left to contend with those incredibly annoying "air stockings" that blow up and deflate at totally erratic intervals, ensuring that neither you nor the circulation in your legs get too comfortable. And let's not forget the random pockets of air that squiggle around your state-of-the-art mattress, keeping the rest of your circulatory system awake and flowing like a mountain stream after a heavy rain.

One more thing: If you're wondering what the best time to mop the floor and empty the garbage in your room is, it's sometime between 4 a.m. and 5 a.m. Apparently dust and germs are caught off guard at that hour.

Now just imagine playing a featured role in that mini-series all day, every day, for a month.

Yes sir, thirty days is a long, long time.

65

... *On the Other Hand*

It seems like only yesterday that it was good that it took forever for 30 days to go by. When we were kids, summers went on for miles and miles and you couldn't see the horizon because it was just too far away. The magic of that last week of school — no work left and the entire summer ahead to just do nothing. When doing nothing meant filling your days with a hundred different things, all of which you did just because you felt like it. That Stuyvesant Town was a grass- and tree-filled sanctuary made the prospect all the more alluring.

The absolute best thing — the thing my friends and I looked forward to the most during those lazy summer days — was convincing the girl of your choice to go into a building with you and make out in the stairwell. It was pretty much a free-for-all, like those National Geographic specials on Sunday night where you get a close-up look at lions battling it out over who would be the lucky one to pair off with the one lioness that was "ready."

The stairs and landings were of corrugated metal that had the look and feel of a waffle iron. If you managed to sit or lie down or do whatever you could manage to do for long enough, relevant body parts were left with the impression of breakfast food; hence the term "waffling" became forever etched on the Stuy Town psyche.

Matty, John and I had a pretty good hit rate back then and managed to spend lots of summer evenings in those stairwells. The only obstacle, other than convincing one of the girls to make out, was actually getting into the building. By 1972, all the entrances had been renovated with lobby doors that actually locked, and residents — grouchy old ladies mostly — leveraged those locks to the hilt to keep horny teenage boys from getting in. But you're gonna have to do a whole lot more than act nasty and say "you don't live in this building" to keep a horny teenage boy away from a stairwell. We used to recruit 10- and 11-year-olds (we were probably 13 at the time) to pretend to be on their way home and follow old people into their buildings, then come back to hold the door open until we got there with our "dates."

This was no small task. This was a covert operation that required teamwork, dedication and skill, and these kids had what it took. They would fight each other over who would be the one to help the "older guys" get into the building, the reward being significant bragging rights the next day: "I held the door open at 15 Oval for Jimmy Cap and so-and-so last night. Snap, he is so cool!" When you're eleven, older kids aged in dog years, so a 13-year-old was *way* older than an 11-year-old as far as they were concerned.

What made the hour in the stairwell all the more entertaining was that the three of us would frequently be there at the same time, on different floors, saying ridiculous things out loud to make each other laugh, while the younger guys would peer over a stairway railing to watch and learn, thinking they were invisible. Matty was the undisputed champ when it came to saying ridiculous shit out loud. He still is. He'll pretty much say anything to anyone. One time when his dad, Julius, was riding him hard about something when he was a kid, Matt couldn't take anymore and sought refuge in the bathroom. But Julius, never far behind, followed him in, cornering him near the toilet, and continued the verbal salvo. God knows what Matt did to make his dad so mad, but boy, Jules was pissed. Out of escape options at that point, Matt decided to go strong. He hocked up a nice fat loogie, spit it into the toilet with enthusiasm, looked up at his father and said "Puhh! That's your mother in there!"

That's your mother in there?? Really? Who says that to their father in the middle of a smackdown? Poor Jules. How does an intelligent, peaceful man even respond to something like that? I'm sure it crossed his mind to stick Matt's head in the toilet to retrieve the loogie, but instead he informed Matt that he loved his mother very much, and walked away.

While Matty, John and I were holding court at 15 Oval, Billy and Tommy were in 522 East 20th Street; Kevin, Brendan and Johnny G. were in 18 Oval (Kevin rivals Matty when it comes to ridiculous, so I may have to rethink my "undisputed champ" statement); and scattered throughout several other buildings were Sean, Bogey and

10 other guys, each one creating lasting memories of their own, which of course we would later share and embellish upon with each other. As a group, we derive great pleasure still in recounting those lazy, hazy, crazy days of summer that helped shape our lives and make us who we are today, for better or worse.

I've always prided myself on my excellent recall, but no one I know has the ability tell a story with uncanny accuracy and attention to detail like Tommy the Wire. Tommy has had a long, successful career on Wall Street, but I believe he missed his true calling. He's one of the best raconteurs I've known, and I've met quite a few. You have no choice but to give in and travel along to wherever Tommy wants to take you once you're hooked. He really should have been a performer of some sort, maybe a talk show host or a circus barker.

While looking for socks or something in my dresser drawer one morning, I came upon an envelope of old pictures memorializing various stages of my existence. I had to laugh when I found a picture of me and Tommy from our eighth grade "dance" performance. For some strange reason we were forced to take a dance class that year, some sort of ballroom dancing, and we (meaning the guys) tolerated it because it was such a convenient way to cop a feel without arousing suspicion. At the end of the year we had the pleasure of performing the various dance routines we had never actually learned in front of our families and friends in the school auditorium.

In the photo, Tommy and I are sporting our "performance" outfits — gray Catholic school uniform pants; a hideous, waist-length jacket with huge, pointy lapels and a cummerbund; a white shirt and a red clip-on bow-tie. It was 1973 and my hair was long, black, and still parted on the side, as I had not yet moved to the ultra-hip middle-part. On our arms are our partners: Anna Leavus, my little seductress for the evening, and Tommy's girl Patricia Fey, both of whom look frightened and confused.

The photo brought back a torrent of memories that needed to be shared immediately. Fortunately, in this age of spy technology, I was able to do just that by simply picking up my Blackberry Bold camera / phone / video / Email / texting / all-access device and snapping a picture of the picture, which I then proceeded to email to Tommy along with a brief note that read "do you recall this very special moment in time?" Tommy's reply arrived seconds later, short and sweet: "I still have the wardrobe. The thing I remember best about that night was that Bogey was a no-show, and you and John convinced Ms. Gherity that I should fill in for him and dance his part with Anne Carlin … sufficiently embarrassed from not knowing any of the dance routine while clasping Anne's sweaty palms, I could clearly see you and John offstage, bent over laughing. I did actually find that amusing at the time. You can plainly see from the picture your stage presence, while I looked scared stiff. Funny that nearly 40 years later, we — and Bogey — would be drinking and playing cards together at 3 a.m. in some country club on Long Island." (Ten of us gathered together recently at a very exclusive country club, played golf, and sat down to a proper jacket-and-tie dinner, after which we proceeded to drink and play cards until 4 a.m. Bogey had been a member of the club for about a month at that point; given how the evening progressed, I assume his membership was revoked.)

Damn, how did those years slip by so quickly? How is it that it's 40 years later and I'm in my fifties now, sticking the Beast with stiff left jabs to keep it off balance, and some of us aren't even around to reminisce and laugh anymore? How is this even fucking possible? I'm really starting to understand why some people just zone out and live in their own little world. How much easier would it be to permanently occupy the spaces in your brain that are filled with everything you're already familiar with and love, like laughing backstage with John while Tommy sweats it out with Anne Carlin, as opposed to stressing out over every little fucking thing. Thankfully, I can upload photos onto my Blackberry Bold camera / phone / video / Email / texting / all-access device, pick up the phone, and relive those moments whenever I need to regain my sanity. I guess the trick is to find that place in the middle where everything is balanced and even: where past, present and future; good, bad and indifferent, all swish together to create peace and allow you to live in the moment. Wow, very Haight-Ashbury of me.

In any event, I was never very good at that:
Been thinkin' about tomorrow

The shades are down and the curtains drawn
All we have is ours to borrow, here today
Maybe all we have is here today

Science Made Simple:
Lesson 2 — The Digestive System (Part 1)

For starters, the stomach is not where you think it is. When you were a kid and you thought you were punching someone in the stomach, that area just below one's navel, more likely you were hitting that poor little Boy Scout in the lower part of his small intestine and maybe catching a piece of his sigmoid colon or his cecum, depending on how far left or right your punch missed its target. The stomach, it turns out, is miles away in abdominal real-estate terms, taking up residence just below the left breast and curling like a "J" into the midsection above the navel, right about where you would expect to find the solar plexus (that other spot kids love to throw punches at). There are all kinds of things going on in there that, unless you've done five years of medical school or been sliced open a few times, it's very difficult to wrap your brain around. The whole thing is incredibly complex.

The colon, also known as the large intestine, is divided into four parts: the *ascending colon*, which starts at the cecum, where it connects to the small intestine and where you'll also find the appendix loafing around, doing nothing productive; the *transverse colon*, which cuts across your abdomen and sits roughly above your navel; the *descending colon* (if you bother pointing out that one part goes up, you're gonna have to expect there's another part coming down, and it too will need a name), which worms its way down the left side of your abdomen; and finally the *sigmoid colon*, which is hardly distinguishable from the descending colon as far as I can tell, but "sigmoid" sounds so cool that they had to throw it in just for the hell of it.

Packed in between all this colonic mass is the small intestine, a slimy blob of connective tissue that looks like a cross between a bunch of snakes frantically mating, and a bowl of chow fun noodles. It is here that the serious business of digestion takes place. This is where the nutrients from the food you swallow are sifted out and diffused into the bloodstream to be distributed to all the other organs and connective tissue in your body that require sustenance to do their job. After the small intestine is done taking everything it needs, it pushes what's left through the cecum and into the big storage tank that is the colon. The colon will use whatever leftover fluid it deems worthy to assist in minor bodily functions here and there (waste not, want not!) and then squeeze whatever shit is left over down through your rectum and out through your anus.

Okay, I suggest we take a little break now because it's too much to digest all at once. (Yes, I know — cheap digestive system jokes.)

Clearly when I was conversing with the O.R. nurse I didn't have the slightest idea what I was in for, but I probably should have. This wasn't my first brush with being prepped for surgery. I was in college when my surgical virginity was taken from me.

I remember Billy coming up to hang out one weekend in New Paltz at the start of my sophomore year. It was early September and the weather was beautiful. I had moved off-campus the previous semester and was living in a housing complex called Riverside Apartments located, oddly enough, alongside a river — the Walkill. It was there that my buddy Leo and I figured out after much trial and error that you could fit exactly one case of Budweiser tall boys and exactly one large bag of ice into a cooler he had lying around, and Billy and I capitalized on that research as we sat down to watch the Yankee–Red Sox game that Saturday afternoon. This wasn't just any Yankee–Red Sox game. This was, as I recall, Game 3 of a four-game series at Fenway in 1978 in which the Yankees, having been down by as much as 14 games to the first-place Sox earlier in the season, were staging a ridiculous comeback and would sweep the series to force a one-game tie breaker in early October for the American League East divisional title. No Yankee fan could ever forget that series, lovingly referred to as the Boston Massacre. Ron Guidry shut out the Sox in Game 3 to record his 21st win. As if that weren't enough, Guidry went on to finish the season 25-3, a Herculean feat, with his 25th win coming against the Red Sox in that one-game playoff at Fenway, the same game in which Bucky Dent, not known as a home-run hitter, hit a three-run blast over the Green Monster in the top of the seventh that put the final nail in the Red Sox coffin. "Bucky Fucking Dent," as Sox fans still refer to him. Who woulda thought?

For a Yankee fan, it doesn't get any better.

After the game, which conveniently enough coincided with the consumption of the last two tall boys, I thought it might be a good idea to get the high-powered BB gun I had recently purchased and go out between the buildings to shoot at some cans. I had done this a couple of times before and it was quite fun. Billy thought that was a fantastic idea, of course, so off we went. After digging a few cans out of the dumpster and setting them up for a sharpshooting contest (because everything has to be competitive), we took a good look around to make sure there were no kids in the area — safety first — before firing the initial round. We were 30 or 40 feet from the targets, but the gun was incredibly accurate because it was powered by CO_2 cartridges — highly compressed air — which made it all the more gun-like.

After about 15 minutes of shooting, which included trick shots like shooting backwards over the shoulder and diving to the ground à la Joe Mannix to roll and fire, someone called to us from a nearby balcony: "Don't you guys think that's kind of dangerous?"

"Yeah, don't worry about it," we responded without bothering to look up.

"I *am* worried about it," the voice continued. "There are lots of little kids that play in this area and you really shouldn't be shooting guns here. Or anywhere, for that matter."

We stopped shooting long enough to size up our nemesis. It was a guy who looked to be in his late twenties, maybe early thirties — Billy and I were 20 and 19 respectively, at the time — and he clearly wasn't going away anytime soon. I thought of firing a warning shot above his head, like Clint Eastwood would have done, and then thought better of it.

"Seriously," I slurred, "I do this all the time and I am well aware that little kids play around here. We're being careful, so why don't you go back inside and let us practice. We're studying to be police officers."

"Are you drunk?" our buddy on the balcony exclaimed. "You're fucking drunk and you're shooting a gun! What the fuck is wrong with you two?"

My patience was wearing thin, as was Billy's, but he was restraining himself, as it appeared I had the situation well in hand. This was not easy for Billy, who is normally quick to react (it's not that he *starts* trouble, it's just that he's not shy about ending it, quickly). That lesson Sister Thaddeus taught us about discipline and restraint back in the fifth grade was sure coming in handy.

Have I mentioned how I hate being told what I can or cannot do? Anyway, who the fuck was this guy to tell me and Billy we couldn't shoot a high-powered BB gun in an area where children usually play after we've polished off a case of beer during a huge Yankee game, as if we didn't know what we were doing and were behaving recklessly?

"Look, I know what I'm doing," I said. "My father's a cop and I've shot guns before. We're watching out for the kids, so why don't you just leave us the fuck alone."

While I was setting this guy straight once and for all, I was mindlessly waving the gun around, completely unaware that it was set to fire because that idiot was distracting me so much. As the words "leave us the fuck alone" found their way out of my big mouth and flew up toward the guy on the balcony, I heard a quick "pffft," the sound the gun made when it fired.

I looked at Billy with a "did I just do what I think I just did?" expression, but Billy didn't notice. He was already looking down at my bare right foot, which had blood pumping out of a small wound down near my toes.

Incredibly, the pellet had missed bone, cartilage and, most importantly, an artery that sat in the general vicinity, instead lodging itself deep within my foot.

I alternated between looking at Billy and looking at the neat little blood-pumping hole before finally glancing at the wise gentleman still positioned on his perch high above. He looked genuinely concerned as he shook his head in disbelief. "Um, do you need me to take you to a hospital?" Mr. Balconi offered.

"No thank you," I said. "I'll just go back inside and see if I can get it out with tweezers."

"I'd go straight to Kingston Hospital if I were you," he recommended. "I wouldn't fuck around with tweezers."

Of course, I had to fuck around with tweezers before Billy was able to convince me to get in the car. *Capa tosta,* my father calls me. It's a Neapolitan phrase that loosely translates to "thick-headed." or "stubborn." He calls me that a lot.

Kingston Hospital was about 20 miles away and my foot was beginning to throb. In an eerie display of classic foreshadowing, I predicted the whole thing should take about forty-five minutes from the moment we walked into the emergency room, to the moment we waved goodbye to all the hot nurses, whose phone numbers would be spilling out of our pockets as we headed back to New Paltz and the many bars that awaited us there. Billy went back to the car to relax with our friend Mary Jane and listen to music while waiting out my "procedure."

"See you in a few minutes," I incorrectly informed him.

Meanwhile, I had decided it would be best to pay for the surgery with cash rather than use my father's insurance. I really didn't want my father to find out, as I was certain that the absurd humor of the situation would elude him. Anyway, how much could it cost to take a little BB out of a foot?

"Are you sure you don't want to submit an insurance claim?" asked the doctor, a proper-sounding gentleman from India.

"I'd like to pay with cash if that's okay," I said. "Will it be more than fifty dollars?"

"Yes, precisely fourteen hundred and fifty dollars more."

"Fifteen hundred dollars for a BB in the foot? I am so dead," I said. It was painful the way the doctor was pulling, pushing and twisting my aching dog as if he were trying to pop the BB out by applying just the right amount of torque, yet I was quite certain that Pops would put me out of my misery with that snub-nosed .38 he wears around his ankle. It wouldn't even pay to make up a story — his cop brain would pick it apart instantly.

Three and a half hours later I was wheeled back to Billy's car by a pretty nurse who clearly had no time for a highly medicated hippie child who had shot himself in the foot and smelled like a saloon. The doctor gave me a prescription for antibiotics, but I didn't bother to fill it. I did, however, fill the one for pain meds. When I went back for a follow-up a few days later, he explained that it was extremely important to start taking those antibiotics immediately: "The wound is already infected" (something to do with the tweezers, I'm guessing). "If the infection continues to advance there will be nothing we can do and we will have to cut the foot off. Your foot is in your own hands."

I can't imagine Billy enjoyed the rest of his weekend visit very much. All I was able to do was sit around with my foot up, popping pain meds that I refused to share. Still, I was glad he was there with me that night at

Kingston Hospital, just as he would be some 30 years later at Memorial Sloan Kettering, along with Matty, John, Tommy, and so many of my friends. My diagnosis, along with that of John and our buddy Bobby Fulham, was a tipping point for many of us, a realization that we might not be invincible after all.

As Gary's much older brother once informed him while attending an uncle's funeral: life is like a giant conveyor belt — it's only a matter of time before you reach the end and plummet into the great unknown. My friends and I are about two thirds of the way along, with a solid third to go if we're lucky. But not all of us have been so lucky. Puhh!

Walter

I should probably take a moment to explain where the expression "Puhh!" comes from and why it's such an important part of this story.

Those of us who grew up on and around Twenty-First Street have a fond but frightening memory of this hulk of a kid named Walter. You couldn't pass by the corner of Twenty-First and First without bumping into him. Walter had Down's syndrome and some pretty serious learning disabilities, but we just thought of him as "retarded" and scary at the time. Back then, those with special needs didn't receive the level of care and assistance they receive today — the result for the most part of widespread ignorance (which in no way excuses such deplorable behavior).

Walter lived in my grandparents' building, so I had the pleasure of running into him more often than most of my friends. His principal means of expression, which he exercised with great authority, was to spit and curse for no apparent reason as you passed by: "Puhh! Fuck you!" It wasn't just the spitting and the cursing that was so startling; it was the particular combination of the spitting and the ultra-aggressive "Puhh" that accompanied it that elevated the act to extraordinary heights. It was an expression of complete and utter disdain.

What could Walter, in his seemingly simple world, have been so disdainful of? Matty and I have pondered that question over the years. Why was Walter so nasty and mean? Why was he so hostile?

One day when I was 12, something happened that offered some insight into the matter, although I wouldn't catch on until years later. I was on my way up to see my grandparents on the fourth floor of their five-story walk-up when I decided it was high time I checked out the roof. I had never ventured past the fourth floor. For one thing, that's where Walter lived. More to the point, there was never any reason for me to go any farther than my grandparents' apartment. On this particular occasion curiosity got the better of me, so I headed north.

On the roof landing I opened the door very slowly, nervous as hell, not knowing what to expect, and wedged a rock in the doorjamb to keep from getting stuck up there for the remainder of my days. I took a couple of steps into this uncharted territory and the first thing I saw, to my dismay, was Walter. He was standing near the ledge, looking down. I thought, "Oh shit, he's gonna toss me off this roof when he sees me." I was about to make a quick exit when Walter turned to face me and I froze. Oddly, he didn't move. He didn't say a word. No "Fuck you!" and no "Puhh!" He just stood there looking at me with a forlorn expression and a combination of tears, snot and drool streaming down his face. I had interrupted what must have been a very private moment for him. And, just like that, he wasn't a scary freak anymore; he was just a sad little kid standing on the edge of a roof, very much alone.

We held each others' gaze for a moment as I tried to figure out whether he had been throwing rocks at people, or whether he was thinking about taking the plunge himself.

"Hi Walter," I finally said in a tentative voice.

"Hi James," he responded in a clear, subdued tone.

I was shocked — shocked that he knew my name, that he could speak so clearly. And he wasn't angry at all, just broken. The poor kid looked so pathetic. Genuinely concerned, I asked him if he was okay.

"Yes," he said with an exaggerated nod of his head, and that was the end of it. After a few more seconds I smiled, turned, and walked away.

I have no idea whether Walter smiled back, nor do I have a clue as to what he might have been thinking. I was just happy to get out of there alive. But I do know that from that moment on, Walter never spit or cursed at me again. Instead, he made a point of saying "Hi, James" whenever we crossed paths. I was so delighted that I was no longer afraid of him that it never occurred to me that all Walter needed to defuse his anger and frustration was a little human interaction, which I inadvertently provided from time to time after that impromptu meeting in the sky. He was aware that he was different and that people treated him differently. And he was devastated by it.

As Matty would later point out, that "Puhh" was Walter's way of telling the world that it could go fuck itself for treating him differently. It was his way of mustering up all the hate and disdain and contempt he suffered and packing it into one powerful little punch to show the world exactly how he felt: "Puhh!"

It is in honor of Walter, who probably never got a fair shake, that I muster up all the hate and disdain and contempt I've come to feel for the Beast, and pack it into that powerful little punch:

"Puhh!" you motherfucker, "PUHH!"

And if Walter were here right now, he'd kick your fucking ass, too. PUHH!

On a Scale of 1 to 10 ...

If you would, try to imagine a large truck, maybe a fully loaded moving van, wedged between two parked cars. One of those cars might be a big SUV, the other a mid-sized sedan (not that it matters). Now imagine the driver of the truck shifting between forward and reverse while flooring the gas pedal so as to continuously slam between the front of one car and the rear of the other.

Do you have that image in your head? Those cars must be in a whole lot of pain, no? That truck has got to be doing some serious damage.

Now, keeping that image in your head, substitute your liver, kidneys, pancreas or any other pair of organs in your abdomen for the two cars. Got it? Good, because when you're suddenly awakened in the recovery room after an extended right hemi-colectomy, that's exactly what it feels like is going on inside your body.

Holy shit! I have to tell you in the interest of being totally open and honest: The pain was so intense I don't believe the word I would use to describe it has been invented. I don't know how long it took for them to pump some pain meds into me after they woke me, but it felt like days. Somewhere in that nightmare I can recall a very nice recovery room nurse barraging me with seemingly nonsensical questions:

Do you know where you are, Mr. Capuano?

What day is it today, Mr. Capuano?

Do you know what year it is?

Who is that standing next to you, James? Do you know her name?

On a scale of 1 to 10, with 10 being the worst, can you tell me how bad your pain is?

Finally, a relevant question: How bad was my pain? Well, let's see. On a scale of 1 to 10, it's a fucking 15 to 20. And I'm pretty sure I made that clear. I do recall demanding that she "make this fucking pain go away immediately."

As for the other questions — Jesus Christ, how was I supposed to know what day or year it was? Didn't the nurse already have that information? Couldn't Dana or one of the technicians have told her? At the time, I had my hands full trying to figure out what planet I was on.

Of course, all she was trying to do was make sure I hadn't slipped into a coma or developed more brain damage than I had when I first went in, but I couldn't appreciate that at the time. She had awakened me after 5+ hours of surgery (just a tad more than the forty-five minutes I had set aside for it in my pre-op conversation with the nurse), during which my good friend Dr. Helm had both his hands inside of me, feeling his way around.

Okay, that didn't sound right. Let me rephrase: It's

routine for surgeons to carefully run their fingers across all your major organs during this type of procedure, just as the O.R. nurse had said, to determine whether or not the disease has spread beyond what they can actually see. In my case, Dr. Helm needed to be extra vigilant because, as I was about to find out, the Beast had been seeding my abdomen for some time with its freakish little clones. There were malignant "lesions" working their way across my small intestine and somehow convincing an alarming number of lymph nodes to let them in as well. Sneaky little bastards.

As the good doctor explained to me and Dana when I was in the recovery room, he was surprised to see this because it hadn't shown up in the CT scans. He broke this news to me in the nicest way after the nurse let the drugs flow freely, so once again in a very loving mood, I let José know this was not something we had talked about before the surgery and therefore he must be mistaken. He ever so gently assured me there were indeed lesions right now marching across my small bowel. As a result, he needed to resect a sizable chunk of said bowel, as well as all the lymph nodes on the right side of my sternum. This was in addition to half my colon being expatriated from its ancestral birthplace.

"Damn," I said. "Is there anything left in there?" Not that I was particularly attached to any of those body parts, but even while stoned I recognized there might be some long-term ramifications to their removal.

riffs that Paul, George and John, in that order, ripped through for 18 measures before culminating in "The End" on side two of *Abbey Road*.

"I don't know," John would reply. "Look at that little bump on his lip. That definitely isn't there on the *Rubber Soul* cover."

"No way man, that's gotta be Paul," I'd holler. "Linda would know. She'd never stay married to an imposter." As I might have mentioned earlier — what dopes.

In May 1976, John and I scalped tickets to see Paul McCartney & Wings at Madison Square Garden during their "Wings over America" tour. We were extraordinarily pumped by the mere thought of seeing a Beatle play live. We bought tickets from the first guy we came across on Seventh Avenue, and had no idea whether the seats were any good or if the tickets were even real. I think we paid 35 bucks each, a lot of money for a 17-year-old in 1976. But boy, it was so worth it. The seats turned out to be amazing, located in the front row of section 110 of the loge (the first tier above the floor seats), and just a bit in front of stage right. When Paul sat at the piano stage left and played "Lady Madonna" and "The Long and Winding Road," he was facing us directly, not more than fifty or sixty feet away. It was inconceivable that we were that close to an actual Beatle performing actual Beatles songs a mere five years after the breakup.

Walking home from the Garden, the two of us discussed every aspect of the show right down to the expressions on Paul's face, both of us certain beyond the shadow of a doubt that Paul McCartney was indeed alive and that the two of us (along with 20,000 other people) had just had the incredible good fortune of spending the last three hours with him.

Now that's the kind of stuff that keeps us moving forward as we swerve to avoid the most menacing potholes we encounter during our brief ride on planet Earth.

*

You and I have memories, longer than the road that stretches out ahead.

– From "Two of Us," by John Lennon & Paul McCartney

OK, James — Time to Go for a Walk

When all the post-surgical confusion began to subside and I found myself back in my room without any recollection of how I got there, the first thing I thought was, "Boy, I'm gonna be lying in this bed for a long, long time." I couldn't even fathom how I would change position, never mind how I was ever going to get up out of the damn thing. "At least the painful part is over," I reassured myself.

And then the nurse came in and announced it was time to get up and go for a walk.

Surely this was part of my post-surgical hallucination. I had heard about this. It takes days, sometimes weeks, for all of that anesthesia to work its way out of your system, and until it does it's impossible to put together a rational thought. Because for a minute there I thought she had said something about me taking a walk.

"You need to get up out of that bed and start walking," she repeated. "It'll help get your organs functioning properly again."

I turned my head as much as I could to see to whom she was actually speaking. Surely it couldn't be me.

Much to my surprise, I was the only other person in the room. "Seriously, did you just tell me to get up and take a walk?" I asked with a small chuckle.

"I did," she replied, "and I don't see what's so funny."

"I'm sorry," I said. "I don't mean to be obnoxious, but you see I just got out of surgery about a minute ago, so you're probably thinking of someone else. Please, don't even worry about it."

"Oh, I'm not worried," she said. "And yes, I am talking to you. Come on, I'll help you. You need to get up out of that bed and start walking."

"There's no way I'm getting up out of this bed. I'll start to bleed or something. Isn't that dangerous? Besides, it hurts way too much for me to move. Just let me lie here a couple of days and then I'll try and do some walking."

"Well, okay, Mr. Capuano. You stay in that bed and relax. And while you're relaxing, your organs will stop functioning altogether and we'll have you back in for emergency surgery by morning."

I was starting to feel a lot less fuzzy at that point and figured I ought to take her more seriously. "I really don't think I can get up out of this bed without going into shock," I said. "I'm in a tremendous amount of pain."

"Look James, I know it seems impossible right now, but I'm gonna help you get up out of that bed and we'll take it nice and easy," she said, much more sympathetically now. "You really do have to walk or complications will set in."

tongue, each of which plays a key role in this process. The teeth chew the food down into smaller bits so that the esophagus and the stomach don't have to work quite so hard. The saliva helps out by contributing enzymes that break the starches down into smaller molecules. The tongue, which can be used for many, many things in addition to aiding in the digestive process, pushes the broken down bits of food through the throat and into the esophagus, where the long journey into the digestive tract begins.

After all is said and done and chewed and swallowed, any material that's left over and for which your body has no use gets stored in the colon and is eventually passed through to your rectum and then out through your butt. Now, granted, some of this is redundant to what we learned in Part 1 of this lesson, but I think it's always important to fully understand how shit happens, so to speak.

*

There's a wide hallway that runs around the perimeter of the floor between the patients' rooms and the nurses' station that doubles as a "track" that everyone uses for these therapeutic jaunts. At any given moment you'll find six to eight post-surgical inmates of all ages hitting that track and jockeying for position. At first it was excruciating and took an hour to struggle my way around once. I remember thinking I was surely obliterating all of Dr. Helm's good work. And I was certain one of those crazy bastards flying around the floor would slam into me at any moment, hurling me back into the operating room. Fucking showoffs.

Fortunately, my friends Meredith and Tony had loaded up a brand new iTouch with gigabytes of my favorite music and surprised me with it one evening. What was really cool was that the iTouch had just come out around the time I was struggling to get back on my feet so not many people had one, making me a standout as I shuffled my way around the track. Tony is a serious gadgets guy, always up on the latest technology. When they finally come out with a teleportation device, I guarantee you Tony will be among the first humanoids to have one; I can only hope he picks up one for me as well.

In the absence of such a device, I was forced to do what all 21st-century humans do to get from place to place: put one foot in front of the other — slowly, methodically, and very painfully. The tunes helped me focus on something other than the excruciating pain that accompanied each step. But each time I made it out there, I was able to go a little bit farther. Before long, I was the crazy bastard flying around the track, showing off. Sometimes I'd even walk counter-clockwise, which was a no-no. Who's sicker than me?

And then the contractions started coming. Every two

to three minutes. My water had broken and I was fully dilated. Now I understand what those four freeloaders I helped create had put Dana through upon entering the world. The nurse was right — walking definitely sped up the re-functioning process, but as my intestines awakened from their slumber they emitted mind-boggling pain throughout my abdomen, doubling me over once again. My friend Felix helped me through the worst of it one evening, but not without a great deal of anxiety, as I'm sure he'd attest to.

I told him repeatedly as though it were all his fault that I should have never gone through with that fucking surgery, that I was worse off now than before. The pain meds did nothing to lessen the pain, my incision was seeping blood, and no one seemed to give a rat's ass. What the fuck did I bother going through with this for?

"Well," said Felix, "otherwise you'd be dead." Good, sound logic.

Felix and I have been friends for a dozen years and have been playing music together for every one of them. Our families spend summer weekends on Fire Island. We were introduced through our mutual friend Mel, who loved to connect people and took great pride in assembling appropriately balanced egos and personalities as though he were constructing the hull of a boat — every last millimeter of cedar needs to fit precisely for it to be seaworthy. It seemed only natural that Felix and I get to know each other, so Mel brought him by my back deck one summer evening. Conveniently, Felix had his guitar with him, and of course the first thing one musician says to another when paths cross and instruments are in hand is, "Hey man, what kind of guitar you got?"

After a minute or two of careful deliberation, Felix opened the case to reveal a gorgeous, blonde-finished, big-bodied Guild F-50 acoustic guitar, with action like butter and an achingly beautiful tone. It called to me like a siren beckoning a lonely sailor. Felix was clearly uneasy as he offered me his muse (you don't just hand a vintage F-50 to any old poser), but relaxed as I proceeded to handle her with reverence, demonstrating that I was worthy. After introducing myself to this lovely vixen, gently fingering her smooth neck and fingerboard to let her know I was no novice (is it getting hot in here, or is it me?), I began playing and singing one of my own songs, a jazzy tune full of sevenths and ninths that I knew would make her blonde wood blush (*"Got to be love, there can't be two ways about it / If there's a heaven above, God knows I can't live without it…"*). I followed that up with a heartfelt rendition of John Lennon's "Across the Universe," and I knew I had her. Evidently this was no less pleasing to Felix, and we've been playing together ever since.

Felix enjoyed a successful career as a recording artist and touring musician in the '70s and '80s, with groupies and everything, having perfected his craft in his home town of St. Louis, Missouri (and when I say "enjoyed," what I really mean is "Holy shit! Tell me another story,

Uncle Felix!") He's played with just about everyone and shared the stage with big-name talent. His most consistent run of success came when he joined the band Angel as their bass player/vocalist. Angel was a hard-rocking arena band that put on BIG shows rivaled in those days only by KISS, the reigning king of the arena show. In fact, it was Gene Simmons from KISS that got Angel signed to Casablanca Records. Legend has it he was sorry he did, never imagining they would launch such a formidable challenge to his own band.

These days Felix has taken it down a notch. Most weekend evenings during the summer you'll find him sitting with me on the back deck in the same two Adirondack chairs that have provided us with unconditional support over the last dozen years, picking and harmonizing and stopping just long enough for a sip of scotch or to puff on a cigar. Quite often people will stop by for a drink and to request a few tunes. Others, like our friend Ricky, bring their guitar and sit in for a few minutes or a few hours. That back deck, late at night, is where my soul lets its guard down to suck in all the harmony it can hold, which I hope will be enough to sustain me through the long winter that inevitably encroaches.

Soup and a Sandwich

It often amazes me how clueless people can be, how completely oblivious they are to what's going on around them. Not just clueless, self-centered. The type that thinks the world is theirs and everyone they come across in it is intruding. Nasty fuckers.

Case in point: While sitting out on the hospital patio one afternoon at a picnic table with our friends Helen and Mike, who had come for a visit armed with two months' worth of reading material for me and a highly irreverent sense of humor, some woman, not a patient, decided that the one extra seat at our table was rightfully hers — if not most of the tabletop. She proceeded to lay her shit out all over the place without so much as looking up to acknowledge we were there. She spent the next few minutes taking stock of her inventory until she set her sights on a little bag with the name "au bon pain" written on it. The four of us sat there watching her in mild amusement, wondering what she would do next.

I was a couple of days out of surgery at that point, feeling like a strong wind could snap me in half, and looking very much like those poor people in the photos the World Hunger Foundation uses when asking for your help in eliminating hunger once and for all for as little as sixteen cents a day. Helen had been making us laugh for an hour or so, a welcome distraction even if it wasn't doing anything for my incision. I was days away from even a nibble of solid food, as were many of my "colleagues" on the patio that Indian summer afternoon. Not that any of this mattered to our table-mate.

Narcissa, as I like to call her, was so wrapped up in herself she never gave a thought to the starving inmates sitting all around her as she fawned orgasmically over her delicious-smelling soup and sandwich. You'd have thought she was the one who hadn't eaten in a month.

Helen, not being one to keep her voice down or her opinions to herself — she used to sell bonds on Wall Street — made it quite clear that Narcissa had crossed the line and was entering the demilitarized zone:

"Is this woman fucking kidding me?" said Helen loudly. "Does this asshole not realize there are people sitting two feet away that haven't put a fucking Saltine in their mouth since the Mets won the World Series [1986, by the way] and she's gonna sit there and masturbate with a fucking deli sandwich?"

While the rest of us howled, there wasn't so much as a hint of acknowledgment from Narcissa as Helen railed on in her best 1980s Wall Street vernacular. This was one of those rare occasions where the danger of busting a gut wasn't just an expression.

To this day I can't look at an "au bon pain" sandwich (or bag) without feeling a nasty stab in my abdomen, and thinking about Helen.

The Control Freak Hands Over the Reins

One of the things I came to terms with during my illness was that my kids are unbelievably spoiled. It's not just my kids; it's everyone's kids. It's amazing to me how within just one generation, going from those who were born in the 1930s and '40s, to those born in the '50s and '60s, parents went from allowing their children to do everything on their own, with little or no parental interference, to allowing their children to do nothing for themselves. My kids can't cut a bagel or plug in a lamp without assistance.

Yes, of course we yell and scream and threaten and punish in order to get them to do what they should do on their own but they know we're full of shit. All they have to do is wait things out for a couple of hours or days and they'll be right back in the driver's seat. And the whole cycle will begin again. And Dana and I will wind up doing everything ourselves like morons because it's less frustrating than having to rely on the unwilling in order to get things done.

How did that happen? Someone should commission a major study on this because it is an incredible phenomenon. I totally get why my parents always looked at me as if I were speaking in tongues when I was old enough to have kids of my own and they'd ask, "What are you doing tomorrow?" and I would inform them: "Nick's got a game at 8:30 but I'm coaching Danny's game at 10:30 so I'll need to get out of there a little early; Brandon's got a party to go to uptown and Jules has a playdate in Stuy Town. We'll probably take them out to eat after that and then to a movie or something."

"When are you gonna have time to relax?" my father would ask with disdain.

"What do you want me to do?" I'd respond. "Should I tell them they can't play Little League or go to a birthday party?"

"Ahh, do what you want, it's none of my business," he'd say, calling an end to the conversation.

When I was growing up, my friends and I could easily go from eight in the morning until eight at night without ever seeing or saying a single word to our parents. They would have no idea where we were or what we were doing. For the most part, they didn't care. If you needed something done and you didn't do it yourself, guess what? It didn't get done. On top of that, you got your ass kicked for not doing it. That seemed reasonable to me at the time. It still does, somewhere in the back of my DNA. And they surely weren't handing out twenty-dollar bills every time we asked for money, as though we were entitled to it. In fact, they weren't handing out anything. If you wanted money, you went out and earned it.

At the risk of sounding like a creaky old-timer who

makes sucking sounds with his dentures, I started working to earn my own pocket money when I was 12 or 13. All of my friends did. I worked at a deli, a dry cleaner, as a receptionist for some Catholic society for the blind, and later on for a cleaning contractor as a maintenance worker in office buildings throughout the city.

The deli was my initiation into the world of the workingman. My brother (already adept at handing out money from his time behind the register at Victory Market) and two older friends, Georgie Janis and Bobby Tudge, worked for Jack, the proprietor of the deli. As Jack was fond of pointing out ad nauseum, I was "the ace from the bullpen, the #1 reliever." When one of those three couldn't make it in, I'd get the call — and I hated it. For one thing, it usually interrupted some extremely important thing I was doing with my friends. For another, I was terrified. I had no idea how to work the counter. I didn't mind restocking the shelves and refrigerators, but having someone ask me for something I'd never heard of when I was working the counter made me a nervous wreck.

"True Blues, please," a gentleman said in an asking-me-to-get-them-for-him kind of way one evening.

"Sure, no problem," I responded, at the same time wondering, "What the fuck are True Blues?" in a mild panic. I didn't have the slightest idea what the guy was talking about but I was too embarrassed to let on. So I started looking around, casually at first, just praying I would spot something with the word "blue" written on it.

I searched under the counter, I looked in the deli case. I glanced at Jack's daughter Gina, a couple of years younger than me, with a pleading expression. While I was scouring the beer refrigerator directly behind the counter for clues, the man finally interrupted. "What are you doing, son?" he asked.

"I'm looking for the True Blues," I said, anxious and confused. "I think we might be out of them."

"Well I appreciate you going out of your way like that, but I doubt you'll find them in the refrigerator," he said. "They're cigarettes."

"Oh, that's right, sorry about that," I said, while Gina stood by the counter, laughing hysterically.

And God forbid kids should ever have a minute of "down time" these days. Every moment has to be structured and planned from the instant they awake in the morning to the moment they close their eyes at night, sleep being their primary escape from the madness. This, to me, is our greatest transgression. There's just no way the mind can entertain a creative thought and follow it through if it's never left to roam free, unencumbered by rules and structure. Never mind that we're creating a generation of robots — there are more serious consequences as well. Youth and rebellion are BFF's, tied together for all eternity. Evolution has dictated the terms of that relationship and the terms are non-negotiable. If kids aren't allowed to break free from time to time and given the liberty to simply "be," they will unwittingly try to cram whatever they think they're missing — the "fun" stuff — into stolen moments wherever they find them. Rebellion and excess becomes the rule, not the exception, because the urge to simply "be" is too powerful to ignore.

Another thing our parents weren't doing when we were kids was sitting around waiting for the phone to ring, or for us to run home crying so they could usher us through every little thing that came up like we do for our kids today. Forty years ago there was no such thing as a "helicopter parent" who hovered watchfully, just in case, and came swooping down in the nick of time to resolve every issue great and small. That was unheard of in my parents' generation.

And you know what? It all worked out just fine for us. We figured out how to be self sufficient. We were hungry and competitive. We learned how to resolve our own issues. In this way, we learned right from wrong. We came to understand the importance of being kind because we experimented with being mean. (You can't be mean today, at least not outwardly. You have to be tricky about it. You can only be passive-aggressive mean.) We learned about compassion and how to help each other, and we did most of it on our own, through trial and error. They let us do things for ourselves back then because they knew what we seem to have lost sight of today: Experience is the best teacher.

Damn, when did I become such an annoying, pontificating old man? Sorry about that.

It took a major illness and a little help from a professional for me to realize (admit) this, but I carried the "self-sufficient" ball a little bit too far up the field. I carried it straight into control-freak territory. I like to pretend it's not the case, but this diagnosis really backed me into a corner and I was forced to fess up:

MY NAME IS JAMES, AND I AM A CONTROL FREAK.

Don't get me wrong — I'm not apologizing for it; I'm simply acknowledging it. There's nothing I can do about it, anyway. It's not like it's by choice. Can I help it if I'm the only one who knows how everything needs to be done, regardless of the area of expertise or subject matter? For instance, I was at a meeting at Goldman Sachs one day with Johnny O and there was a rather intense discussion going on concerning the pros and cons of high frequency/automated trading, which relies on powerful computers and ultra-complicated software code to execute trades at lightning speed. After about 15 minutes, I jumped in during a pause to inform the geniuses in the room that while "I really don't know very much about this stuff," I felt compelled to speak. And, of course, I spoke. Goldman Sachs! What's wrong with me? (Three years later, the cons became readily apparent when the Dow Jones Industrial Average lost 50 percent of its value within a matter of days as machines ran amok. I only wish I had accidently said something about the potential for *that* to happen during my off-the-cuff treatise.)

have?

In much the same way (but for different reasons) that my parents allowed me to do things for myself and learn from each experience, I had no choice but to watch as everyone around me picked up the pieces and started doing the things I thought only I could do. Life went on without me having to do everything myself. I wasn't indispensable after all. That's a tough lesson for a control freak to learn.

Just in case you're wondering, I've forgotten it already.

Avastin, Oxaliplatin, Fluorouracil, Leucovorin and Scotch

What's that all about? Jeez, I don't even know if I can do this one justice, but I'll try. Let's see: It's about walking up to the schoolyard bully — the sonofabitch who has been tormenting you and everyone you know since the second grade — with four big-ass, kung-fu motherfuckers by your side, and in front of the whole school taking him by the neck with one hand, putting him up against the lockers and saying loud and clear for everyone to hear: "Bitch, if you so much as look at me the wrong way again, if I so much as hear you whisper my name in passing without genuflecting on one knee, if you happen to be walking on the same side of the street as me and neglect to cross to the other side, I will wreck you. I will make you wish you never laid eyes upon me or even caught a glimpse from a distance."

Does that make sense? Let me put it another way: It's about walking through a pack of hungry wolves in the middle of the night with your pet grizzly bears at your side and ten pounds of steak in your pocket, and giggling as the wolves make room for you to pass, with their heads down and their tails between their legs. It's about looking the devil in the eye and saying, "Don't even think about it, Red. Puhh!"

agents as a more efficient, less destructive way to obliterate our enemies. (Why blow up and destroy perfectly good buildings and infrastructure when it's just the people we want to fuck up?)

Because the Beast was already in the advanced stages of neutralizing my existence, it was crucial that Dr. Keltner concoct a formula that would hit the little shit with maximum impact out of the gate. The right mix of chemicals at the exact dosages was needed to save my ass from extinction. As it turns out, Avastin + Oxaliplatin + Flourouracil + Leucovorin + Macallan 18, multiplied by the Power of Will, equaled Kryptonite over the Beast. The formula looks something like this:

$$\frac{(A+O+F+L+M18)\ PoW = K}{B}$$

It's a potent cocktail of chemicals designed to hit the bastard from all angles, cutting off its food supply and shriveling it up like the Wicked Witch's legs under Dorothy's house (another scene that terrified me as a child).

It's a very aggressive, very powerful chemo combo we're talking here:

- **Avastin**, the newest, most recent FDA-approved member of the team, cuts off blood supply and prevents new blood vessels from forming to feed the tumor (now, *there's* a nice, old-fashioned word for cancer; what's with all this "lesion" and "disease" crap?).
- **Oxaliplatin** is a platinum-based anticancer drug that seeks out and destroys cancer cells (you go, Oxaliplatin!).
- **Flourouracil**, a protein inhibitor, gets inside the cancer's DNA/RNA and disrupts production of the bad cells so they don't multiply as efficiently.
- **Leucovorin** is not a chemo drug but a vitamin complex that enhances the effectiveness of Flourouracil.
- **Scotch**, well I think we all know what that is. I took it upon myself to add 18-year-old Macallan, my favorite single malt, to the mix after several rounds of treatment. Having experimented with it for many, many years pre-cancer, I had reached the inevitable conclusion that it makes me feel good. Real good. (I'm not sure the doctors will agree that it's okay to augment treatment like this based upon this type of research, but hey, I'm a risk-taker.)

Side effects? Shit yeah! Plenty of 'em. But this is where the rubber meets the road and you get to step up and captain the team. This is where you utter inspirational phrases like "no pain, no gain" and "what doesn't kill you makes you stronger."

And you know what? The side effects are wonderful. Horribly, miserably wonderful. It's all about perspective. You have to learn to embrace the side effects because while you're enduring them, the cancer is having fucking conniption fits, writhing in pain while the poison strangles the living shit out of it. And then it dies.

Keeping it dead can be challenging, but I'm a glass-half-full man. Plus, I'm alive. So from my perspective, living with these inconveniences for a year was well worth it. Side effects? Bring 'em. I'll take that shot all day, every day.

In a nutshell, here's how this special chemo combo side-effected me, in descending order of misery:

➤ neuropathy, a numbing of the hands, feet, fingers and toes (painful but bearable if you don't mind tripping over yourself and constantly spilling your coffee);

➤ extreme sensitivity to cold (I had a full winter's worth of treatments so this one sucked);

➤ constant nausea (not enough to make me vomit, but enough to let me know it was there, constantly);

➤ exhaustion (treatments have a cumulative effect, so the more I got, the more tiring);

➤ metal mouth (really hated this one because everything I tried to eat tasted like gunmetal, whether steak or pasta. And you have to eat or you won't regain your strength, the quintessential Catch-22);

➤ raw, sore throat (makes it hard to swallow gunmetal-flavored food);

➤ mild headaches (just annoying, really);

➤ elevated blood pressure; watery eyes; dry, cracked fingernails and skin;

➤ no real hair loss on my head, but a thinning of body hair (who cares);

➤ short-term memory deficit and general confusion (been that way since 1973);

➤ various other nit-picky things.

Most of these side effects completely subside within months after treatment ends. Some stick around longer (neuropathy, sensitivity to cold, confusion and irritability, possibly short-term memory deficit but I can't recall), but don't really get in the way of normal, day-to-day functioning. There's other stuff that gets in the way of that, believe me when I tell you.

Matty often accompanied me to treatments, largely because he would do anything to get out of the office, but he had other motives as well. He figured that if all his friends were getting sick (by now, Herbie had gotten in on the non-Hodgkin lymphoma thing, but he kicked its ass, too), it was only a matter of time before the Beast came knocking on his door. What the fuck, maybe he could sweet talk one of the nurses into slipping him an ounce or two of chemo, not a lot, just a prophylactic dose, enough to ward off disease. He entertained the staff quite a bit with this modest proposal, but what they didn't realize was that he was half serious. Maybe more than half.

The Flourouracil was administered over a 48-hour period via a tiny pump. On one end was what looked like a baby bottle filled with a yellowish liquid that hung from a loose belt around my waist; on the other end, a thick needle that was fixed into the septum of my subcutaneous infusion port, located in my upper right anterior chest wall. (I could throw in another Science made Simple installment here, but I'll be brief: The needle was stuck into a port implanted under the skin on the upper right side of my chest.) Ports are commonly used for long series of treatments. It's convenient, and it keeps your veins from collapsing. On the other hand, it was incredibly uncomfortable to walk around and sleep with this thing connected to me for two days at a time. Worse, you had to go to an authorized dealership — a hospital or infusion center — to get it disconnected when it was done infusing, and disconnecting your pump isn't the top priority of the nursing staff. Understandably so, but you could wait for well over an hour to be freed from this unnatural attachment. Fortunately, my friend Tracey is an oncology nurse at Sloan Kettering. She was more than happy to make a house call and disconnect me in the comfort of my bedroom. Her husband, Ray, thought it only fair that if Tracey got to spend time alone with me in my bedroom while I had my shirt off, similar privileges ought to be afforded him with Dana. Shit, I thought; the least I could do under the circumstances would be to support his position.

Eventually, Tracey taught me how to disconnect the thing myself (I guess she got bored). Poor Raymond is still waiting for Dana to come through on her end of the arrangement. Good luck with that, Ray. I'm pulling for you.

Oh, I Get By With a Little Help from My Friends ...

I am unfortunately fortunate enough to have had several friends beat me to a cancer diagnosis — some by a lot, some by a little. Each of them played a substantial but slightly different role in my cancer education and subsequent ability to cope with my diagnosis and treatment. To a considerable degree I have these three guys, as well as my friend David "Otis" Russell, to thank for keeping me moving in the right direction. (When diagnosed with oesophageal cancer six months before my diagnosis, Dave held my hand and guided me until it was time for him to bid us adieu.)

When I look back on all of this, it's as if I had been in the Beast's waiting room, trying on different coping mechanisms, seeing which one fit best.

Of course, nothing is ever a perfect fit. In the end, I took a little from each of them.

Stephen

Usually when you insert the prefix "non" before a word it has a positive connotation. For instance, if you say someone's "critical," more often than not it means they're fucked, but if you add the prefix "non," everyone breathes a sigh of relief: "He's on the *non*-critical list now, Mrs. Johnson. Your husband is going to be just fine!"

So why is it that when the doctor comes out and says "Mrs. Johnson, it's just as we thought, your husband has non-Hodgkin lymphoma," Mrs. J shakes her fist toward the heavens and screams, "WHY GOD, WHY???"

What the fuck? "Life threatening" or "non-life threatening," which would you pick?

Stephen was diagnosed with non-Hodgkin lymphoma in 1998. That's the bad kind. Apparently, regular old Hodgkin disease is preferable if you have to have one or the other.

I know Stephen had the "bad" kind because that's the one that killed Jackie O. and King Hussein of Jordan very shortly after they were diagnosed. Stephen, fortunately, managed to dodge that bullet and even hock a nice, fat loogie on it as it flew past his nose. Puhh!

The news of his diagnosis came as a shock. How the fuck could he have non-Hodgkin Lymphoma? He was only 39. He paved the way for me to understand what cancer and subsequent treatment means to the person who is actually diagnosed. After a painful biopsy, he didn't have surgery, but he had radiation therapy five days a week for five weeks, complemented by several rounds of chemo. It was an all-out blitz. The poor guy didn't have a minute to breath, but he handled it like a champ. He never complained, just spoke with humor and honesty about what he was going through both physically and mentally. He's a natural mentor. He showed me that it's okay to talk openly and directly to people about what you're dealing with because, for one thing, they want to know but are afraid to ask; for another, talking about it actually helps you get your head around it.

Stephen still gives quite a bit of his time to survivors and recently diagnosed patients, helping them learn to relax and get a handle on what's going on.

John

In spring 2004, John was diagnosed with colorectal cancer — more "rectal" than "colo." Within a year, it had taken up residence inside his lungs as well. It was on the move, Stage IV.

I'm not sure what the makeup of John's cancer was, but neither was he; he wanted as little information as possible. While Stephen devoured information and used it to help get things straight in his head and inform those around him on a need-to-know basis, John pretty much closed his eyes and prayed that when he opened them again, he would find it had all been a bad dream. I'm not making a judgment, because people handle a cancer diagnosis their own way. It's all relative.

When John realized that a firm grasp of the details

would do nothing more than hinder his ability to cope, his wife, Marie, picked up the ball and carried it up the field for a full five years without ever looking back. Marie and John had been together since the eighth grade, and Marie knew him better than anyone. (Yup, he finally found the nerve to ask 13-year-old Marie Frey for a date, right after Patty finished kicking his ass. They were married a decade later. At some point they had melded into a single entity — a dual-brained, single-souled organism — and they couldn't be happier.)

John was several years ahead of me in his diagnosis and I watched closely as he and Marie did their best to domesticate the Beast. Through the fear, the anger, the discomfort and multiple procedures, John kept his mask on, allowing all but his closest friends to believe everything was just fine. He maintained his uniquely ridiculous sense of humor throughout, but I knew it was a struggle. Marie became medical researcher, record keeper, adviser, nurse, cheerleader and psychologist. She had each and every conversation with the doctors and fed back to John only the info she felt he was able to swallow — and in small, pre-digested bites.

"How can you not want to know what you're dealing with?" I asked John during one of our "what do you think happens when you die" talks. "Wouldn't it be helpful to know a little about what you're up against?"

"Jimmy, I don't need to know the specifics about what's going on," he replied. "I just need it to go away."

"I know it totally sucks, and I'm so sorry you're going through this, but it is what it is and you have no choice but to deal with it," I stoically informed him. (This was prior to my own diagnosis, so it was easy for me to be brave.)

"Oh, I meant to ask you," he said, "do you or any of your cousins know how to run background checks on animals? Tiny birds in particular. It's a long story but I'm running into problems that a little foresight might have helped me avoid." (This is a classic example of John's absurd sense of humor, which I find hilarious. It's also a classic John way of misdirecting a conversation.)

As for the "what happens when you die" bit, that's a topic he and I had been ruminating on since we were kids, and not at all exclusive to his (or my) cancer diagnosis. We came up with a convoluted theory involving reincarnation, quantum mechanics (with a focus on multi-dimensional string theory), Freemasonry, the Beatles, Frye Boots, and tiny birds. I'm not yet ready to publish our findings; when I do, I won't be surprised if those Nobel people came a-knockin'.

John approached his dilemma from the "ignorance is bliss" school of thought, the only problem being that he wasn't ignorant, and bliss was nowhere to be found. He happily guided me through my treatments, having already experienced similar, and helped me stay focused and strong. He was always so good at helping others with their problems; it saddens me deeply that he had such a hard time affording himself the same courtesy.

Mel

Mel, the guy who introduced me to Felix, was diagnosed in the summer of 2004. Though sixteen years older than me, Mel was a confidant.

He spent his entire working career as a biologist, teaching at the prestigious Stuyvesant High School in New York City. As a biologist, he would have nothing to do with pedestrian cancer diagnoses like colo-rectal or non-Hodgkin lymphoma. Mel went large — Mel went brain cancer. The sonofabitch hit him where it hurt, right in his giant fucking brain. Glioblastoma, the baddest of the bad. Life expectancy for someone diagnosed with this is typically 12 to 18 months. Mel had 12 months to come to terms with his sentence before he slipped into a six-month slide, but he made the most of it.

He was a realist. He didn't pussyfoot around with sentimental bullshit. It's not that Mel was without feeling; on the contrary, he loved his family and friends deeply, but was more acutely aware of how our big brains and deep thoughts were a bonus, not an entitlement. "In evolutionary terms, we're really nothing more than freaks of nature and we should learn to appreciate our unique circumstance for what it is," he would say.

Although sidetracked by two invasive brain surgeries (is there any other kind?), he bounced back enough to reconnect with those he loved, and in doing so taught us

The Plan

As nice as all that poisonous, systemic infusion stuff was, I felt like I was still missing out on something. Surely there was some other torture I could endure to spite the Beast, to really beat it down. If only there were something else I could do. Oh, wait — I still had that second surgery to look forward to! Goddamn, how could I forget? Another sneak peek inside to see if any of those damn lesions were still hanging around. So I still had that going for me.

What Team MSK had in store for that sonofabitch beast in Round Two would make it pine for the good old days. Actually, it would make *me* pine for the good old days, but hey, what doesn't kill you makes you stronger, right? (Told you that would come in handy.)

Round One, in which JH debulked me (that sounds so dirty), took place September 7, 2007. My "second look" surgery happened five months later, on February 14, 2008. "Second look" is as invasive as the first peek except that, fingers crossed, I wouldn't have to endure another extensive debulking. That would have presented a real problem because Dr. Helm had already taken out as much small intestine as he felt he could safely remove, with no choice but to leave some disease behind. More than half my colon was gone. (I hate to say it, but I'm really starting to miss those chunks of large and small bowel he took out.

The lymph nodes a little bit too, but not as much. I didn't think I would, but shit, we were together 48 years.)

For Round Two, the hope was that Dr. Helm would simply slice me open again, take a good look around and feel up every last millimeter of my small intestine. (I'm an inches and feet guy myself, but doctors love all that fancy medi-metric speak). Then, for fun, he would have a go at what was left of some neighboring organs, stuff everything back in, and break out his trusty Swingline to close me up again. He planned to re-enter through the initial incision, the one that had recently healed and still hurt like hell, but at least I wasn't going to end up with railroad tracks all over my abdomen.

Best-case scenario: another week to ten days in the hospital, including prep, surgery, a little healing — and my favorite part, where we make the Beast pine for the good old days. That's when the doctors make good on the special plan we'd been discussing since shortly after my first surgery. Because there was some disease left behind, it was *molto importante* that they continue to treat me as aggressively as possible, so we déjà vu'd our way through the surgery and the post-op and the 15 to 20 on a scale of 1 to 10 and the walking and the yada yada yada. Now it was time to execute.

When Dr. Helm walked into post-op to see how I was doing this second time around, he had much better news for me than he did the first time we performed this part of the act together. "Jimmy, you're not going to believe this," he said, giving me one his giant, generous smiles. "I spent a long time feeling around your abdomen" — he really seems to enjoy that for some reason — "and there was no sign of disease. And I mean I checked everywhere. That is one benign abdomen you've got, my friend."

Wow! How amazing was that? I hadn't dared allow myself to believe the cancer would have been obliterated this time. Apparently, Dr. Keltner's formula really smoked those lesions. My body had responded extremely well to the therapy. "No sign of disease anywhere." Ho-lee-shit!

Dana and my father were also in there with us, of course, and wore equally gigantic smiles on their faces.

My father, by the way, is kind of like Zelig. He has this ability to show up wherever he wants and no one ever dares question or say a word to him about it. In hospitals, I've noticed, he effortlessly takes on the appearance of a wise old physician. I'm pretty sure he could have walked into the operating room and handed Dr. Helm a scalpel. Maybe he did, for all I know. It's truly fascinating.

Anyway, one minute we were all looking at each other, grinning like fools, and the next, I was back in my room with my trusty old morphine pump dripping away. It was reflex at that point to push the button every 10 minutes to release one or two drops of the precious serum. It's set up that way so you can't overdose on it. The thing I found most interesting was that an outside company provided the distribution of the morphine and that every time you hit the button, the cash register rings at their headquarters. I, or my insurance company, was being charged by the drop. I only wish I had come up with that idea first. It's always so fucking obvious after someone else does it.

There I was, back in my room, wondering if Dr. Helm had really said what I thought he said or if I was hallucinating again, when I reached up to scratch an itch on my lower right ribcage and found a gigantic lump. It scared the shit out of me until I remembered why it was there. When Dr. H opened me up, he implanted a second, much larger port up around my rib cage. Sutured to my ribs, in fact; most unpleasant. It was about three times the size of the first port and had a long tube that snaked through my bowels and was left open on the downward side (there's a lot of "snaking" involved in cancer treatment, I've noticed). As nasty as that sounds, the reason for that tube being there is much nastier. Believe me.

*

So, what the fuck is this plan I keep referring to, right? I was just getting to that. Jeez.

The "plan" involves pouring chemo directly into the abdomen. This is a process known as "intraperitoneal chemotherapy." Sounds repulsive, yes? That's because it is.

It has to be. You can't fight the Beast with sticks and stones and hope to break its bones. It'll just keep coming back. You need heat-seeking missiles that are big and nasty enough to wipe the fucker off the face of the earth. In a word, you need poison.

Science Made Simple:
Lesson 5 — Marinating the Beast

There are two ways to douse the Beast with poison. The first is Hyperthermic Intraperitoneal Chemotherapy (HIPEC — although I still can't figure out what that "E" stands for; maybe that's the secret sauce), which is administered in the operating room in conjunction with a good old-fashioned debulking (cytoreduction surgery). It can take on average eight to ten hours for both procedures, which is an awfully long time to have your guts hanging out. While you're opened up on the operating table, after they've cyto-reduced you, the doctors connect you to a machine that circulates heated chemo fluid throughout your abdomen for several hours, making sure it gets into every little nook and cranny before they drain it off. You're out cold during this hyperthermic event, and thank God for that. Apparently, when you heat chemo to a certain temperature (107.6 degrees F, or 42 degrees C), it's able to kill the bad cells while leaving most of the good ones alone. (Fahrenheit vs. Celsius; millimeters vs. inches — can't we just pick a system and stick with it?)

I opted to go with the alternative method of delivering this torture, known as EPIC: Early Post-Operative Intraperitoneal Chemotherapy. Here the chemo is poured directly into the abdomen through the implanted port soon after surgery is over. Instead of getting siphoned out, it gets "absorbed." All this would prove to be far more challenging than the horrible HIPEC.

The reason for administering the treatment this way is that sometimes cancer cells don't attach themselves fully to the blood stream, particularly within the abdomen. They just kind of float around freely until they find a spot they like and then acquaint themselves with the neighborhood. If they really like it there, they stick around and invite their friends. Before you know it, they've taken over. All you need is a single, minuscule live cancer cell to repopulate the entire block with illegal alien cells. Pushy little fuckers.

It's difficult for systemically infused chemo to reach them if they're not in the bloodstream, and it's impossible for the doctors to detect them in sub-microscopic form. When researchers and doctors realized how effective intraperitoneal chemotherapy could be they began to use it more broadly. This was wonderful news for those of us who were diagnosed within the past eight to 10 years, as it meant another weapon in the arsenal, a powerful one at that. Cancer cells love to roam around the abdomen, and it wasn't until some medical research genius figured out that if you pour chemo directly onto them, you can administer higher doses with fewer side-effects (because it's so localized). They first used this procedure on women with ovarian cancer, as well as on those with rare forms of cancer of the appendix.

In my case, my disease was a confounding mix of classic adenocarcinoma, the most common form of colon cancer, and, my doctors believe, some sort of appendiceal cancer, likely of the carcinoid variety, and which had apparently "spewed" some baby-Beast-bearing mucous into my unsuspecting gut (you have to pay a little more for cancer this special, but I knew a guy). To complicate matters, the cells were poorly differentiated, which meant they bore little resemblance to the cells from which they originally mutated, making it more difficult to determine the most effective course of treatment.

When Dr. Keltner originally spoke to us about doing the HIPEC therapy in conjunction with the "second look" surgery, we were limited as to venue. Several places out of state had experience heating up and killing cancer cells, but it meant spending a week to 10 days in yet another hospital even farther from home. It would have been too disruptive for my already weary family, so I asked if there was any other way we could do it.

"We could actually do it here," said Dr. Keltner, "but it would be on an outpatient basis and take quite a bit longer to complete the regimen. Also, the chemo does not get heated in this instance."

"Will it have the same impact?" I asked.

"Additional time in treatment is typically beneficial," he said. "Of course, nothing is guaranteed, but I recommend you participate in the program. Dr. Helm could easily implant the second port during the surgery; he's done it many times before."

I still wasn't sure I wanted to go ahead with The Plan, as I knew I still had plenty of systemic treatment ahead. But after speaking with knowledgeable family members who practiced medicine, as well as Dr. Fuks (especially Dr. Fuks), I realized that I didn't have much choice. I was going to have nice, room-temperature chemo baths on local turf. Just as well that the decision was essentially made for me because I'm not much of a gambler. My gambling is generally limited to what some friends and I partake in on "steak night."

Years ago, five of us decided to embark on a systematic tour of every steak house in the city, not stopping until we had hit each one at least once, including new ones as they sprang up along the way. We take turns picking the venue, which in and of itself is a gamble whenever it's Tom Ryan's turn to choose. Our squad consists of Adam, our point guard; Tom, our 2 guard; me, at small forward; Jordan, our power forward; and KT, our center — who if not for his disproportionate height would be better suited to play towel boy or equipment manager. It turns into a very expensive evening for the loser of the first-round wager, as he has to pick up the tab for five guys who like to eat a lot and drink good wine. The "loser" is chosen via an entertaining and nerve-wracking game known as Credit Card Roulette. At the end of the meal, each of us puts a credit card into a napkin, and the waiter puts the napkin behind his back, shuffles the cards, and slowly draws them out one at a time. Last card out loses.

In all the years we've been playing this preposterous game, Adam and KT have been the most consistent winners — as in, they don't have to pick up the tab. It's like winning the lottery, except backwards, kind of. Personally, I've fared rather well, but not as well as those two. Meanwhile, Tom and Jordan have borne the brunt of the pain, particularly Jordan. It's at the point where it's a serious bummer when Jordy loses because he's always so devastated. I even suggested via email before our last outing that we forego roulette and split the bill evenly because Jordan was no doubt going to lose his house and act like a bitch the rest of the evening. Jordan, not being one to take an insult lying down, immediately retaliated with insinuations and accusations about our wives, leading to a continuous stream of replies, each funnier than the last (and all of them unprintable).

So, who do you think lost the game and had to pay for the meal that night? Jordan, of course. He immediately started to complain, but we abused him so heavily that he had no choice but back down and participate in Round Two of the games, known simply as "Pink or White." At least this would give him the opportunity to win back some cash. Unfortunately, Jordan's luck with Pink or White is about as good as it is with Credit Card Roulette.

Pink or White is a simple game of chance that requires no skill whatsoever. It's based entirely upon good fortune and the benevolence of the gaming gods, who evidently hate Jordan. We each take a pink packet of Sweet'N Low

I was fresh out of second-look surgery when Dr. Keltner decided it was time to start the infusions. I'm talking 24 hours fresh. My incision was once again seeping blood, I was in excruciating pain because I'd become way too tolerant of my morphine dosage and they refused to increase it, and the second port Dr. Helm had put in hurt like a sonofabitch. Stick a big, thick needle into it now? I don't think so. Bathe my raw, tender abdomen in poison for a few days? Just try motherfucker; just try.

I thought they were kidding (again), but I was wrong (again). These people do not fuck around when it comes to trying out all their cool new cancer-killing techniques. The non-thermal chemo baths I was about to take consisted of a three- to four-hour visit to the infusion center every other Tuesday, Wednesday and Thursday for three months, during which my friends in white coats filled my abdomen with Fluorouracil and God knows what. They poured in two litres on Tuesday, another on Wednesday, and a fourth litre Thursday (I'm a quarts and gallons guy myself, but there's no sense arguing). That's four full litres over the course of three days. Translation: That's a lot. Picture one of those big plastic bottles of soda — I think they hold two litres. Imagine having that entire bottle poured slowly into your abdomen through a long straw. Now imagine substituting an even deadlier, more brutal form of poison than soda. Do that for three days in a row, while you're fully awake and fully aware. It's insane. Your body doesn't know what to make of it because it's so foreign and unnatural, and your poor brain is trying desperately to pretend you're in the Caribbean, enjoying sand and surf.

The staff didn't seem to think it was too big a deal. They'd seen this before and the side effects weren't supposed to be as bad as with systemic treatments, but who are they to judge? Have *they* had four litres of poison poured into their abdomen on a regular basis?

After each infusion was completed, I had to lie in the bed and turn myself 90 degrees every 15 minutes like a pig on a spit to make sure the chemo penetrated my entire abdomen and thoroughly marinated every bit of tissue residing there. The chemo actually hurt the outside of my organs, if you can imagine that, and the pain was accompanied by this bizarre bloated feeling that stuck around for a week at a time. You literally feel like your abdomen is going to explode. That's why they schedule it for every other week — it would be physically impossible to do it weekly. This isn't the kind of bloating like when you drink too much beer or eat too much pasta. That's inside your stomach. This goes on throughout your abdomen, so not only are you aggravating your stomach, but also your kidneys, liver, large and small intestines, pancreas, lining of your belly, and anything else the chemo comes in contact with. It's something you have to experience personally to fully appreciate, although I hope you won't try that just to try to prove me wrong.

I scheduled my treatments for late afternoons so I could go to the office at least a few hours in the morning. Obviously, the company couldn't function properly without me. I struggled through each Wednesday after the two litres went in because I'm selfless that way, then barely made it to the office Thursday, and there was just no way by Friday. The real miracle here was how the company managed to survive.

It took a full week for the poison to be "absorbed" and work its way out of my body, during which time I was constantly dry-heaving. Doing that with a fresh, eight-inch incision in your abdomen is a very bad thing. I was also growing more concerned that not doing the systemic treatment for three months — the treatment where the chemo is infused through the bloodstream — would allow the bad cells to regenerate, so I bothered Dr. Fuks yet again and he was kind enough to explain that the chemo was being partly absorbed into the bloodstream as well. It was like having the best of both worlds. Or the worst.

In hindsight, the first round of infusions at the hospital was my least favorite. I had no idea what to expect and was still incredibly sore from surgery. I called Dr. Fuks one evening during the first off-week (the poor guy never should have given me his number) and said, "Zvi, I know this chemo wash thing is supposed to be really beneficial and all, but I have to tell you there's absolutely no way I'll be able to do this for three months. I'm going to tell Dr. Keltner when I see him this week that I'm done. We can just go back to the systemic treatments and do those for a few extra rounds."

"Right — now you're an oncologist," as Roy would

say.

By now you've gotten a sense of what Zvi Fuks is like, and you'd be hard-pressed to find someone more generous. I truly love the man. But no one, and I mean no one, tells Zvi anything. You are free to make a suggestion, or to phrase something in the form of a question, which sometimes works. But you do not tell.

Zvi's response to my little tantrum was simple and direct: "Listen to me, Jimmy, if I thought this treatment would only add a slight benefit to your chance of recovery, a small percentage in your favor, I would tell you there's no point in making you suffer needlessly. But I strongly believe this treatment will add greatly to your ability to survive this ordeal. You're young and you're strong and you're just going to suck it up and go through with the entire regimen. You'll thank me later. Do you understand what I'm saying, Jimmy?"

Did I understand? Did I have a choice? The moment he put "strongly" and "greatly" in the same sentence, I knew I was done. I was going to do exactly what Zvi told me to do. And I've been thanking him for it every day since.

As with anything new and promising in the field of medical research, intraperitoneal chemotherapy is not without its share of detractors. There's not enough empirical evidence that the risks of this aggressive and invasive procedure outweigh the rewards. But three years after I endured it, I'm sitting here typing this story on my laptop. That's all the empirical evidence I need.

Whenever anyone asks my opinion on whether they should put themselves through this medieval torture, I unequivocally tell them yes, they should. I did this recently for my friend Julie, one of the bravest people I know. I also make sure to tell them to expect the worst and not to be surprised when their old conception of "worst" starts to look pretty mild by comparison. It's fucking awful. But when you're at the point where doctors recommend intraperitoneal chemotherapy, it's probably the best shot you've got at sticking around long enough to memorialize the experience in a memoir.

149

Psychological Torture, Plain and Simple

During the first year of your sentence (as in: "I sentence you to a year of hard treatment"), you meet formally with your medical oncologist every three months or so. The purpose of this meeting is to review how well you are responding to treatment, whether or not an adjustment should be made, how you are handling the side effects, and, most important, to evaluate your latest CT scan. This last part is where a fresh new torture comes into play.

Forget water boarding, electric shock and bright lights. Child's play! If the authorities are truly desperate to get information out of someone, all they have to do is tell the person you detect some late-stage colon cancer. Next, give him a CT scan and have him wait a week or so for the results. At this point he's well on the way to a nervous breakdown. The clincher is when the nurse escorts him into the oncologist's examining room while uttering the words "the doctor will be in to talk to you shortly" as she closes the door behind her.

Then make him wait. Two minutes. Five minutes. Ten, twenty minutes. Holy Shit! It must be so bad even the oncologist can't face it!

By now, the patient is so completely out of his mind

that he'll fess up to anything:

Q: "Did you break into that apartment last night?"

A: "I did, I did."

Q: "Did you rip off that deli?"

A: "I don't know what I was thinking."

Q: "Did you leave that backpack full of explosives in Times Square?"

A: "Yes, and I am *so* sorry."

Q: "Did you shoot Abraham Lincoln?"

A: "How did you know?"

The only other thing I can think of that even comes close to producing this kind of breakdown is to lock a person in a small room with my friend Sean for an extended period of time. Trust me when I tell you that this person will quickly give up his or her firstborn to make Sean stop. Throw in Kevin for good measure, and there's not a being on the planet who can withstand the psychological abuse. These two will wear anyone down.

Sean works in the film and television industry as a First Assistant Director (as well as some other lofty positions), and has worked on lots of major motion pictures and television series, as has our director friend, Johnny Gallagher. (I'm not name-dropping, I'm just bragging about my friends a little bit. If I wanted to name-drop, I might tell you that I've spent a fair amount of time in the company of Academy Award winning actors Susan Sarandon and Tim Robbins over the years; that our sons played baseball together; that their son and his band once wrote a song called "Danny From My Baseball Team," and that Susan is as sweet as can be — a great mom, very down to earth and not at all impressed with herself. If I were to tell you stuff like that, *then* I'd be name-dropping.)

In one of the movies Sean worked on, he was also cast in a small role that perfectly illustrates my point regarding successful interrogation tactics. *For Love of the Game* stars Kevin Costner (whom I've never met, but Susan and Tim know him from their *Bull Durham* days, which technically takes six degrees of separation down to, like, one degree). Costner plays an aging major-league pitcher named Billy Chapel, who needs to prove himself one last time before he throws in the towel. In several of the stadium scenes, you can clearly hear a lone voice in the crowd relentlessly heckling poor Billy. He's so loud and abusive that he gets under Chapel's skin. In a role he was born to play, Sean is actually listed as "Heckler" in the end credits.

AssBelly

It's so comforting to have the support of your good friends while you're going through the most traumatic event of your life.

Mid-August on Fire Island. I'm standing at the surf's edge with Kenny, Michael, Brian Power and Yaron. (Yaron is Dr. Fuks' son; it's through my relationship with him that I was fortunate enough to become friends with Zvi many years ago). It's a beautiful day –sun shining, sky a deep blue, the kids entertaining themselves for a change. I'm feeling about as good mentally as I'd felt in a long time. I am nearly at the end of my treatment, and I have already started to put weight back on. Maybe even a little too much weight.

My normal attire for the beach is one of those longish bathing suits and an old buttoned-down work shirt. (I tend to retire my old work shirts to the beach when they're no longer suitable for the office. I highly recommend it. They're lightweight and loose, and unbelievably comfortable, minus all the starch. Just roll up the sleeves and you're good to go.)

So I'm standing down by the water with my good friends and I say, completely out of the blue, "Have I shown you guys my tragically disfigured mid-section yet?"

"No," they say, *ensemble*, clearly not the least bit interested in even a glimpse.

"No, seriously, you gotta check this out."

So I lift up my lightweight, incredibly comfortable work shirt and pull down the trunks a little to show off my brand new, hemispherical mid-section.

As you can imagine, once you've been gutted and stapled closed a couple of times, you've got a pretty good seam working. It begins to take on a life of its own. At this point, the extra weight I've added is making me more self conscious. When you put weight on, even a little, with a tight crease down the middle of your belly, it gives the impression of two separate and distinct hemispheres. The more weight, the deeper the crease.

So I'm standing there after spending the last eight weeks trying to work up the nerve to take off my shirt in public when Brian looks down and without the slightest hesitation, on a beach full of sunbathers, hollers: "HOLY SHIT! YOU'VE GOT ASS-BELLY!!!"

So much for removing my old work shirt on a crowded beach, or anywhere, ever again. From this moment I will forever be known by my Native American handle, "AssBelly." I will be called this by my good friends "Short Man Who Can't Surf," "Was Better Looking Forty Pounds Ago," "Dopey Irish Bastard," and "Arms like Gorilla." (To be fair, "Short Man" could easily have been called "Motherfucker Can Ski" if he were in a friendlier tribe; chicks still dig "Was Better Looking," irrespective of girth; "DIB" would probably still be known as "DIB" regardless of tribe; and "Arms" … well, he's a highly respected, Grammy Award-winning record producer, so he's got that going for him. BTW, I have witnessed Gorilla Arms at work in the studio. It's an amazing sight. He can be sitting down, fiddling with some low-end decibel tweaks on track one, and without ever having to get up from his chair or move his body reach all the way across the board to track 48 and nudge a fader down on a background vocal without missing a beat. It's definitely an advantage having extended brachia when mixing a potential hit record.

After the Thrill is Gone

Here's something crazy for you: There's a kind of thrill that goes along with the fear and uncertainty of a late-stage diagnosis. Granted, my initial reaction wasn't, "Boy, this is kind of exciting," but as I wandered a little farther down the road, it hit me:

There's something about being in the general vicinity of death that brings you back to life.

It snaps you right out of complacency. Suddenly every thought counts, every action. You can't put off until tomorrow anymore. Things became crystal clear and my focus so sharp I could have slayed the Beast with just a glance. The survival instinct becomes overwhelmingly strong; I couldn't fight it if I wanted to.

I suddenly found myself in a club I never truly understood. Sure, I had heard the rumors about people who have been diagnosed with cancer developing this strange kinship with each other that no one else can understand, and now here I was on the other side of the fence, knowing rather than wondering about it. I'd been on a whirlwind tour for months with a bunch of strangers who knew exactly what I knew, felt exactly what I felt. We shared a common experience that enabled us to look at each other and telepathically signal, "Yeah, I know."

And we *did* know. We drew strength from and

encouraged each other through simple eye contact. Those other "strangers" who were there day in and day out — the crew at the front desk in the lobby, the admin staff, the nurses, doctors, technicians — every one of them let me know with a kind word or a smile that I wasn't alone. They were right there with me. There was safety in numbers. This misery so loved company.

Mind you, none of this talk about bonding with strangers is meant as a slight to any of my friends or loved ones, without whom I couldn't have made it this far. I truly believe things would have progressed differently without the positive energy and love they sent my way for a full 525,600 minutes. But there's always room to let others in. The heart has a limitless capacity.

I was so familiar with the disease after a while that I started to feel like we were contemptuous old friends (my "survival of the fittest" instincts kicking in). We became intimate. I got used to having it around. I could even turn my back for a little while and not worry. There was an army of people waiting to pounce should the old bastard try anything funny.

One day I found myself in the examination room (my "Room 101" for those of you familiar with George Orwell's *1984*), a year or so into it, awaiting the results of my first post-treatment CT scan. This was the big one. The moment of truth.

"No change from your last scan," Dr. Keltner announced matter-of-factly (even though he was secretly excited for us all). "There's still no evidence of disease. Treatment's done and we won't need to see you again for another three months."

There they were — the magic words I'd been waiting to hear. Un-fucking believable. I was done. I was good. I kissed Dana, we both hugged Dr. Keltner, and all was right with the world.

On the way home the light went on: *What does he mean I won't need to come back for three months? Who the fuck is gonna take care of me until then? This is bullshit!* Yes sir, euphoria turned right around into panic in an instant.

That's when the real struggle began.

Wait, Isn't This Supposed to be the Happy Part?

My rational self considered "no sign of disease; don't come back for three months" music to my ears. Psychologically and emotionally, it was nails on a chalkboard. The good news sent me on a slow, steady, psycho-emotional tailspin and there was apparently nothing I could do to stop it.

I couldn't sleep. I'd wake in the night to torturous thoughts that were having a kegger in my head. Rather than get up and try to distract myself, I'd lie there trying to get back to sleep, which was about the worst thing I could have done. Being alone with my thoughts was no longer a good place to be.

Eventually I turned to meds. Ambien CR: time-released sleeping pills, a six-hour nightly reprieve. I couldn't sleep — or cope — without it.

Meanwhile, I shared the seemingly fantastic news with everyone. "Yup, cancer-free! Can you believe it?!?" I was genuinely excited to let everyone know because it clearly meant so much to them. They were at the end of an incredibly stressful year.

I, on the other hand, had been coddled, pampered, and handled with care since diagnosis. I had been Nero, fiddling, while Rome burned for everyone around me. Sure, I was hard hit at first, but everyone rallied and took much of the weight off my shoulders. Other folks' cancer diagnoses bring out the best in people.

Now the poles reversed, an incredible phenomenon. While everyone around me could finally let down their guard down and get on with their lives, I went the other way. I wasn't so tough anymore. I was alone. What the fuck was I supposed to do now?

I never spoke a word of this out loud. There was no way I was going to be ungrateful in the face of this gift. It was my shit to work through, and I was an expert at that.

The control freak resurfaced. It was time to get myself in gear.

So I got on with my life. I slowly fell back into my normal routines: I was coaching fall travel ball again, albeit less enthusiastically. I was back at work full time, though not at full strength. We had just moved from Stuyvesant Town to Gramercy Park and were in the process of settling in. People stopped treating me like I was a wounded puppy (which was a shame, because I really enjoyed all the petting). Days and weeks went by and I began to realize it wasn't going to be as easy as I thought to just "get on" with things, but I certainly wasn't going to bother my family with any of this. It wouldn't be fair to them. My friends would surely abuse me. Nope, I'd get through this on my own. It was time to move on.

I tried. I really did. At the very least, I didn't think anyone had noticed my new-found dilemma. I'd be at my parents' house on a Sunday watching the Giants with my dad and my sons, and my mother would badger me constantly, asking me what was the matter. *"Nothing,"* I'd say. "Would you please stop asking me that?"

Dana too was relentless: "I know something's wrong, so why don't you just tell me?" she'd ask, and I'd answer, "Jesus Christ, why do you keep insisting something's wrong? What's wrong is that you keep asking me what's wrong. I'm fine. Can't you just leave me the fuck alone?"

Wait, let me think this through. Give me a moment to regroup. Let's see, the top three presents on my all-time Christmas wish list were neatly wrapped and sitting right in front of me, just waiting for me to tear into them:

1) I'd just been given the green light by the guy to whom I'd entrusted my life;

2) My treatments were D-O-N-E- done;

3) A miracle had just occurred, and I was the undisputed beneficiary.

What the fuck? Was I out of my mind?

One day while my entire family was at my parents' apartment for my mom's birthday, a setting in which I would normally be quite content, I noticed everyone was talking, laughing, eating, and having a great time. Everyone but me. The Giants had just scored on the Eagles following a perfectly executed drive that ate up about seven and a half minutes on the clock, and the room erupted. While the guys in my family were busy high-fiving each other, I sat in a daze, oblivious to everything going on around me, struggling to keep the demons at bay.

The one thing that did register, however, was the look on my mother's face. I caught a brief glimpse of it from across the room. It was as though the cone of silence had descended from the ceiling and come to rest around me at one end of the room, and around my mom at the other. Everything went quiet in that moment and I could actually hear her say without moving her lips: "I caught you, and you know it. Something's going on and you'd better tell me what it is." It was just a look, but it forced me to acknowledge that something was actually wrong. Very wrong. Once I acknowledged it, I could no longer turn away.

When I finally spoke to a doctor, I described it as "black cloud" depression. I'm sure that's not a clinical term but it's apt nonetheless. (I'm petitioning to get it into the Physician's Desk Reference, so don't you try taking credit for it.) There was an impending sense of doom hanging over me all the time, and all I could do was sit around and wait for the imminent collapse. Surely I would lose everything. My family would be devastated. I would live in misery the rest of my days, which probably wouldn't be too many, since it was only a matter of time.

I was sitting on my couch one Sunday afternoon trying

to watch *The Godfather Part II* on some cable channel (a futile effort because, for one thing, there was a commercial every 45 seconds; for another, I was completely unable to focus) when Dana started in on me again. "Seriously, what is going on with you? Something's not right. Are you sick again? Just tell me."

That's it! I suddenly realized that they thought I was acting like this because I must be sick again. I was so caught up in my own head that I had no idea how my crazy behavior was affecting anyone else. I have a habit of keeping bad news to myself and Dana has a habit of overreacting (there's a pharmacy's worth of potions in the linen closet just in case one of the kids sneezes), but I knew at this point the jig was up.

"I'm not sick again," I said. "I'm just incredibly depressed and I have no idea why."

"THAT's all that's bothering you?" she said. "I thought you were going to tell me you felt another tumor or you were bleeding when you went to the bathroom. Are you fucking crazy? After everything you've been through, you let something like that get to you? Go see a shrink. Make an appointment. Sloan has an entire facility to help people like you. They'll probably prescribe an anti-depressant and you'll feel better in a few days. Go make an appointment right now."

I guess if you're secretly worried that your husband's cancer has come back and you're on the verge of having people refer to you as "the widow," it's a relief to hear he's simply suffering from depression. Of course, if you're the depressed husband, relief isn't quite as easy to come by. But for the second time in a year, I followed Dana's orders without putting up a fight and I made the appointment (my grandfathers, while undoubtedly appreciative, must be rolling in their graves). Within a week I was standing in an elevator at 641 Lexington Avenue hitting the button for the seventh floor, on my way up to meet my newest, bestest friend, Dr. Steven Presley.

Dr. P

Being a control freak means I'm always right, so I had never even entertained the thought of seeing a psychoanalyst. What could a stranger possibly tell me about myself that I didn't already know?

I had no idea what to expect as I stood at the receptionist's desk waiting to be noticed. Now that I was actually here, I was a little annoyed with myself for being talked into going so easily, so I was playing around with different approaches I might take with this guy when I met him so that my hour wouldn't be a complete waste. Maybe I'd just sit quietly, staring, waiting for him to ask me questions, which I would then answer in noncommittal ways: "Yes, I suppose," or "I guess," or "Sort of." I could throw in a "You tell me, you're the expert." Yup, I'd show this guy I wasn't some little bitch he could just pick apart with his fancy Ph.D. and comfortable chair.

"Do you have an appointment, sir?" asked the receptionist, snapping me out of my trance.

"I do," I replied.

"Please fill out these forms, and Dr. Presley will be with you shortly," she said in a pleasant enough way.

Shit! If there's one thing I'm bad at, it's filling out forms. I get hung up on the simplest questions: "What is the insurer's Group Number? What is the insurer's ID Number?" What the fuck is the difference? Were they asking me for the one with the 27 digits, or the one with the 16 digits followed by a dash followed by some letters and then some more numbers? I've never gotten it right. I'm even worse with driving directions. If there's a wrong turn, guaranteed I'll take it, even with GPS. I'm pretty sure the GPS woman, that sweet voice that gives you audible directions, knows it too. I swear I can hear her voice get a little louder and less patient as we approach a turn or an exit she knows I'm about to miss. One time, I'm pretty sure I heard her whisper "fucking moron" under her breath as I sped past my exit.

After muddling through the "new patient" form, I looked up to find Dr. P approaching. He looked like a good enough guy, around my age, but I wasn't about to just cozy on up to him and tell him my life's story. He'd have to earn that. He was going to have to prove himself worthy of taking me on as a project. I was considering telling him I needed to use the restroom and then bolting as soon as he turned his back (oh, yeah; clearly I don't need any help). Then I thought about simply explaining to him that I had made a mistake — that I really didn't require psychoanalysis, I was just doing this to placate my wife. She's the one who needs some fucking psychoanalyzing.

On the short walk down the hall to his office, I thought to myself, "What the fuck is wrong with me? I have a problem and this guy can more than likely help me fix it. I mean, he specializes in getting fucked-up cancer survivors back on track. Is this really a good time to start acting like a major-league asshole?"

I quickly realized that sitting down and having stream of consciousness conversations with a trained, objective third party was neither threatening nor intrusive. A good one simply steers you toward uncovering for yourself the roots of all your evils. If you complement those conversations with a daily 300 mg dose of Wellbutrin (or an equivalent mood stabilizer), the road to recovery may very likely open up before you and beckon you to take the wheel.

It's not quite as automatic as that. When I first sat down in Stephen Presley's office — which, by the way, had the most uncomfortable chairs I've ever sat on — I wasn't sure how to get things rolling, so I just opened the floodgates.

"Stage IV, colon, cecum, Avastin, depressed, cancer's gone but what if it comes back, my kids, I know it'll come back, everything sucks, everything's great, I'm so confused."

On I went. It was a Google search gone bad. I went from "You'll never break me, motherfucker" at the reception desk to "I'm such a pussy, please help me Doc" in a few seconds time.

"Whoa, let's slow down a little here," said Presley. "We can talk about whatever you want, but let's take things one at a time. You'll get it all in, I promise."

We talked about everything. Whatever popped into my head was fair game and worth exploring: my fears, my strengths and weaknesses, my frustrations, the disease. Everything.

Example: Particularly disturbing to me was my new-found inability to multitask. I've always been very good at juggling lots of things at once without getting frazzled, and now I could barely do one thing, let alone a bunch. I was easily confused and frustrated. I had no patience for anything. Commotion of any sort sent me into a tailspin (still does). It was affecting my performance at work. For a while there, I was literally hiding in my office with the door closed, praying no one would walk in and ask questions or make small talk. My behavior was affecting Dana and the kids, too.

"Yeah, you try having fucking cancer and see how *you* act," I'd blurt out to no one in particular. It was the anti-me, and I wasn't enjoying it either. To top it off, I was relatively certain I was turning into a paranoid-schizophrenic.

"We call that Chemo Brain," Dr. Presley said. "We haven't done enough clinical study on it yet since it's a relatively new phenomenon, but it's real. We see it all the time."

"You mean there's actually a name for it and other people have it too?"

"It's pretty common," Steve said. Yeah, by now he was "Steve." "When you think about it, it's not a stretch that all the poison you were bombarded with wreaked havoc on the chemical composition of your brain. You're all out of whack."

"Wow. That makes total sense. I'm chemically imbalanced. Will I eventually get my shit together?"

"We don't know yet," he said. "We'll figure that out over time. But there are behavioral modifications we can suggest in the meantime to help you deal with your symptoms."

It was Dr. P who finally got me to own up to my "dictator" aspirations. I spent long, leisurely sessions describing how stressful my life was while recounting the scores of wonderful things I do for my family, conveying it all with a thinly veiled "can you believe how great I am?" undertone.

"You know, you're doing a real disservice to your family," Steve said one day.

I was flabbergasted. "How do you figure?" I said. "I just explained to you that I'm completely selfless when it comes to my family and you're telling me that I'm doing more harm than good. What sense does that make?"

"For one thing," Steve said, "you're denying them their own sense of accomplishment. Depriving them of the simple joy of achieving things on their own. Do you plan on being there five, 10, 20 years from now, still doing 'everything' for them?"

"Of course not, that's ridiculous," I said.

"You're right, it *is* ridiculous. But how do you suppose they'll figure out how to do things for themselves if you never let them do things for themselves?"

I had assumed they would learn by watching me, the same way far less intelligent monkeys and lion cubs do it in the wild. "Classical conditioning, I think you guys in the psych department call it," I said, throwing it in Presley's face.

"Type A obsessive-compulsive behavior is what us guys in the 'psych department' call it when referring to human beings," he responded. "Are you sure you're not doing all this to satisfy your own needs? That maybe you're being a little too controlling?"

"Yeah, well, I'm responsible for them," I rationalized. "They can't do things for themselves nearly as well as I can do them. This is not about me. You think I actually want to live this way?"

"Left to your own devices, I don't think you have a choice," Steve said. "It's the way you're wired. But you really need to take a step back and let others do some growing. The same way you did when you were going through your physical recovery and had no other choice. Did the world fall apart then?"

I fucking hate it when other people are right and I can

no longer out-argue them.

Thanks to Steven Presley, I began to see a glimmer of light. Granted, light can travel a long, long way in a pitch-black tunnel, but it was there. And I felt like I had just taken my first step toward it. There was an end in sight. It may take days or weeks or months, even years, to get there, but there was an end in sight.

*

For tomorrow the sun will rise; and who knows what the tide will bring?

From the movie *Cast Away*

The 7th Precinct:
A Nice Place to Visit, But ...

There's something very special about celebrating your 50th birthday, along with the one-year anniversary of your cancer-freeness, with four of your closest friends and some 17-year-old Puerto Rican kid you met in a holding pen at the 7th Precinct. Very special indeed.

Let me start at the beginning so you can get the full gist of my idiocy. My friends and I have a tradition of getting together at least once every summer for a "sleepover" at my place while my family is away. A fair number of these guys moved to the suburbs while their kids were too young to abuse them for it, so we don't get together en masse nearly enough anymore.

The evening usually starts off with a serious meal involving moderate alcohol consumption, followed by a whole host of shenanigans involving excessive alcohol consumption. I say "usually" because we sometimes skip the meal and go straight to the shenanigans, etc.

This particular August get-together was more festive than previous sleepovers for a couple of reasons: I had just turned fifty that July. We were all slapping the ass of the half-century mark (give or take a smack), but my 50th coincided with the one-year anniversary of my cancer remission. My treatments had ended the previous August and my most recent CT scan confirmed I was still cancer free.

It was a bittersweet celebration, however, as John would have just turned fifty too, had he not succumbed to the Beast the year before. Marie had the foresight to throw him an extravagant 49th at SPQR in Little Italy with 200 of his closest family and friends. Roger McTiernan, funny bastard that he is, lamented in his toast to John: "What is it with these I-talians? Who throws a big 49th birthday bash? They must know there's a hit or something coming so they wanted to squeeze it in."

Poor John, there was a hit coming alright. He lasted another eight weeks after battling that motherfucker for five years (the cancer, not Roger). I still cannot comprehend that he's not here anymore. It doesn't make any sense. Fucking cancer. PUHH!

With that in mind, and what with my Chemo Brain and that fucking black cloud still hanging over my head, it didn't take much to get me from pleasant get-together with the guys to a holding pen at the 7th Precinct at two in the morning — as Officers Fatfuck and Ramos can attest to should they refer to their little notepads.

We kicked off the evening at Matty's with some scotch, wine and plenty of food from Carmine's that Matty paid for and I stopped to pick up on the way over there (nice move on my part, picking up the food after it's already been paid for). Billy, Tommy, Jimmy McDevitt and I all went straight there after work, and there was little doubt we'd be in for an evening of laughs. Matt lives with his wife, Gigi, and their boys Jack and Luke in the same penthouse apartment he grew up in, the one where he spit in the toilet and called it his dad's mother. His gigantic terrace is one of the nicer places in the city to sit, eat and drink on warm summer night.

Jimmy, as usual, brought over some ridiculously expensive wine and a nice bottle of scotch, so it didn't take long for us to get loose. We spent two or three hours eating, drinking and abusing one another when Jimmy started to get the itch. Having grown up in Rockland County, he was sure he'd be missing out on something if we didn't show up at whatever the latest hot spot was at the time, pretending we were still twenty-three and wondering why the real 23-year-olds looked at us like we were their fathers.

Jimmy and Tommy met when they roomed together at Oneonta State University freshman year and Jimmy has been an indispensable part of the crew ever since. He decided we should head to the Lower East Side. Until recently, that was one of the last places you'd want to hang out at two in the morning, but in New York City neighborhoods change overnight, and this was, according to Jimmy, the place to be in the summer of 2009. The Meatpacking District, while still full of great restaurants and bars, was getting old and it was time for another rundown, hooker- and drug-infested neighborhood to have its day.

We took our time getting there, stopping at random bars and clubs along the way. We even stopped at this wacky little burlesque place that was desperately trying to recapture the glory of the Roaring Twenties and failing miserably. After sucking down a quick round at the tiny little counter they were trying to pass off as a bar, I noticed that Tommy had disappeared.

"Where the fuck did he go?" I wondered out loud.

"I haven't seen him for about ten minutes," Matt said.

"Probably in the bathroom," Jimmy joined in.

It was Billy who set us straight. "Turn around and have a look up at the stage," he said. "That boy clearly didn't have enough toys as a child."

There onstage was Tommy, dancing behind some scantily clad, drastically overweight entertainer who appeared more than a little frightened by her new partner's spontaneous choreography. While the rest of us howled, the bouncers and pretentious twenty-something patrons debated whether to beat the shit out of us. The bouncers would have been a problem, but the twenty-somethings didn't have a shot. For one thing, Matty is like a fifth-degree black belt, and Billy's overhand right is justly famous. We'd all had our share of bar brawls and "rumbles" with our neighbors from Alphabet City in the early '70s (Alphabet City spans Avenues A, B, C and D from Houston through 14th Street, and is more commonly referred to today as "The East Village"). A few years earlier, there would have been punches thrown for sure. Fortunately, we've matured. We managed to find the exit on our own and continue on our way. One crisis averted, another to come.

McDevitt was intent on taking us to "Hotel on Rivington," the hot spot du jour. The rest of us didn't give a shit and would have been happy to go home, since we'd already been drinking for the last six hours, but we didn't have the heart to deprive him.

First I need to describe what Rivington Street was like before its renaissance, and I use that term loosely. Dana taught fourth grade in the New York City public school system for a number of years, many of them at PS 140 on Rivington and Ridge streets, four blocks from where we were now headed. She taught there from 1985 through 1989, and it was an adventure every day. She never knew what she was going to walk into as she headed south on Ridge.

One morning while she was about a block away, she saw lots of activity by the school's front entrance. As she got closer, she realized there were 10 or 12 alleged drug dealers face down on the sidewalk with another dozen or so NYPD detectives standing over them, Glocks in one hand, cuffs in the other, informing them of their "rights" — as if they should have any. The cops had been using Dana's classroom for surveillance purposes the prior week, keeping a close eye on the crack den in the abandoned building 20 yards away. While they were busy staking out drug dealers, Dana had been busy conveying to her students the importance of memorizing both the multiplication table and their Miranda rights. It didn't even faze those kids. They were used to it. On a field trip to the 7th precinct (yes, the same place that factors into this chapter later), the kids were being lectured by the desk sergeant when two detectives brought in a guy in cuffs, and one of the little girls looked up and said with a big smile, "Hi, Uncle Jesus!" Then there was the time young Angel brought a butter knife to class because he was going to "stab my friend Antoine." Before taking Angel to the principal, Dana had a brief conversation with him that went something like this:

Dana: "Angel, what are you doing with this knife in school!?"

Angel: "I'm going to stab Antoine for saying shit about my mother."

Dana: "Okay, a) we don't curse in school, and b) what did we say about stabbing our friends?"

Angel was 9 years old at the time. You can't make this shit up.

That should give you a pretty good idea of what the neighborhood was like before "hot clubs" began to spring up. So now picture five middle-aged, neatly dressed white guys, with Jimmy McDevitt in the lead, arriving at Hotel only to find dozens and dozens of twenty-somethings waiting outside, desperate to get in. Ludicrous. We immediately informed McDevitt there was no way we were standing on line to get into this place. Young James McD., always full of frenetic, nervous energy, assured us he would straighten it out with the guy at the door. Meanwhile, the rest of us sat on the stoop of a building across the narrow street to enjoy the entertainment he was about to provide.

While watching Jimmy frantically wave his arms and push his hair back while talking at warp speed and getting absolutely nowhere with the guy, Billy decided to walk around the corner to a bodega (an Hispanic mini-mart) for a six-pack of beer. There we sat, content for now with our cigars and our beers, bothering no one, when a patrol car pulled up. In New York, the open container law is strictly enforced. You're not allowed to have an open container of alcohol in a public place or you get a ticket and the city gets some revenue. Depending on the mood and intelligence level of the cop, and whether he has anything better to do, you can then be hassled for any number of other minor things.

For a few minutes we thought they weren't going to bother with us because they weren't in any hurry to get out of the car. But then Fatfuck emerged with his giant 25-year-old gut out in front, and with Officer Ramos close behind, both of them looking all tough and authoritative as they approached the scary-looking, nicely dressed, middle-aged, birthday-celebrating guys to demand some ID "from all a ya's," to quote Fatfuck.

Okay, not the way we had planned on winding down the evening, but we figured they'd just give each of us a ticket and we'd move on. Not a big deal. Fatfuck and Ramos went back to their car and proceeded to do whatever it is they do with IDs while making the alleged perps sweat it out. However, I am a veteran of "Room 101" intimidation tactics, so all this served to do was drive up my blood pressure. As we sat on the stoop waiting, Jimmy ran across the street under cover of darkness to toss the evidence — our cans of beer — into a trash can, which gave us all a good chuckle.

It was twenty-five minutes before the two officers decided it was time for a second round of browbeating. They were gonna show these entitled Wall Street motherfuckers just what acting out in their jurisdiction was gonna get them. They asked a few bullshit questions in tough-guy voices and walked back to the car to make us wait some more. (By the way, none of us are entitled anything. We all come from hard working middle-class families, and we've all busted our asses to get to where we are today, and we're working harder than ever to maintain it. You don't know when you're on the rise that getting there is the fun part. Once you get to a reasonable level, all you do from that point on is worry about how you're going to stay there, because while your earnings may increase moderately your expenses go up exponentially and the two are never in sync again. Getting ahead is impossible; keeping up is the best you can hope for. It's funny, surviving cancer hasn't magically changed my perspective on any of that.)

I couldn't sit there any longer while these idiots kept us waiting so I approached the car very respectfully and let Officer Fatfuck know that we were sorry if we got carried away, that we were celebrating a medical milestone for me. "Officer, I'm sorry, we should have known better," I said. "I've been pretty sick, and making it to my 50th birthday was kind of a big deal." Then I shared with him that my father is retired from "the job" and that I have lots of family and friends who are still cops, and that if he could move things along it would be appreciated because we had to get up early in the morning for work.

Back in the day, if you were the son or family member of a cop, you maybe got your hand slapped but you were let go immediately for a stupid little thing like this. But you know what Fatfuck had the nerve to say to me? "Go back over there and sit on the stoop until I tell you to get up." To which I replied in utter surprise, "What did you just say?"

"You heard me," he repeated. "Go back over there and sit on the stoop until I tell you to get up." Then he rolled up his window and dismissed me.

I happened to look down and notice the "CPR" slogan on the side of the car. "CPR" allegedly stands for Courtesy, Professionalism and Respect. Well, there was no C, no P, and definitely no R coming out of that patrol car.

"Are you fucking kidding me?" I screamed. No

reaction from Starsky and Hutch, so I banged on the window again. That little jerkoff, who was young enough to be my son, rolled the window down a couple of inches and just looked at me. "Are you fucking kidding me?" I repeated a little louder. "You're a disgrace to that fucking uniform."

So what did Five-0 do? He rolled the window back up and dismissed me a second time. I returned to the stoop enraged.

"Will you shut the fuck up and sit down?" Billy said. "You're making shit worse now. Let's get our tickets and get the fuck out of here."

Too late for that, I thought to myself. I was well into it with chubby at this point.

In my entire life, I have never been in trouble with or even the slightest bit disrespectful to a cop. We were all part of the same family. When I was growing up, one cop looked after another cop's loved ones without having to be asked. The way these two were acting was so outrageous I almost spit on their windshield. (I said "almost," in case you missed that.)

I went back to the stoop, where Fatfuck and I eyeballed each other for five minutes while I kept pointing at my watch and mouthing very slowly and deliberately, "Hurry the fuck up." This only served to make them take even longer doing whatever it is cops do while sitting in their cars, making you wait.

Another twenty minutes had gone by when Tommy needed to use the bathroom. Jimmy suggested he let the cops know where he was going, and Tommy reluctantly walked over to the Fatmobile and informed Fatman he'd be right back — he was going to use the bathroom in the bar across the street. "No you're not, get the fuck back over there and sit down," said the wannabe tough guy. "What? Fuck you!" replied Tommy the Wire, and he and Jimmy proceeded down the street to take care of business. Once again, no audible response from the antagonists in the car.

I couldn't take any more of this, so I made another pilgrimage to the window and reminded New York's finest that they were still douche-bags and an embarrassment to the force, and still fucking this and still fucking that, until Billy and Matty convinced me with some level of force to sit back down and shut the fuck up. Tommy and Jimmy returned a few minutes later (long enough to have a quick beer at that bar, I realize now as I write this), and the five of us sat there, annoyed as hell, waiting to break free and salvage what was left of our sleepover.

It was well over an hour before an NYPD van pulled up behind the patrol car and five more cops jumped out, ready for action. Those douche-bags had called for backup! The seven of them huddled on their side of the street developing a plan for subduing the dangerous, middle-aged, birthday-celebrating white guys who had been caught drinking beer on the other side of the street. After going over who was gonna do what, they made their approach. For some reason, the five new guys were each holding one of our driver's licenses. One at a time, they informed the owner of the license just what the infraction was, as well as the value of the ticket: twenty-five bucks. After a wasted hour and a half, and the work of seven uniformed cops, we collectively we owed the city $125.

"You kept us sitting here all this time for a $25 ticket?" I asked, just to be clear. "And for that you two with your guns and your tough-guy attitudes had to call for backup? And you're not embarrassed? You two are fucking pathetic."

I couldn't stop myself, nor did I care to. A couple of the new guys were clearly sorry they'd been dragged into this nonsense and made a point of telling us so, but the others were gung-ho to hassle us as much as possible. They were probably trying to incite us so they'd have reasonable cause to search us, hoping we were carrying massive amounts of cocaine. If you get enough big drug busts you get your gold shield. I could see the next morning's headlines: "Fatfuck and Ramos nab Middle-aged Urban Professionals for Possession of Large Quantities of Cocaine: 'Not on my beat!' Exclaimed Officer Fatfuck."

I couldn't leave well enough alone. I started in on the two of them again in front of their friends. I was on them pretty good, leaving them little choice but to shut me down somehow. I was encouraging them to consider a career as crossing guards when Officer Ramos decided he had heard enough. "All right, you've got your tickets, now it's time to move on," he said.

"Move on?" I exclaimed. "Now you want us to move on? What if we don't wanna move on? Maybe we want to sit right here and smoke another cigar, jerk-off?"

I guess the "jerk-off" sent him over the edge because the next thing I knew, he had me up against the wall with my hands behind my back. I know he was pissed because he made the handcuffs so tight that after a minute or so, I no longer had any circulation in my fingers.

At this point, and with a full crowd of twenty-somethings enjoying the show, I segued into a diatribe on police brutality, which is how I wound up in the back of a patrol car that night. Now, I don't know if you've ever been in the back seat of a police car, but I gotta tell you, it's not built for comfort. There's about four inches between the back seat and the divider in the middle.

"Do me a favor, pull the front seat up a little so I have more room," I told them.

I'm extremely claustrophobic and I knew right away that this wasn't going to work for me. There was no way I could deal with being jammed into the back seat with my hands locked behind my back, but I wasn't about to let Crockett and Tubbs in on that or they would have driven around the Lower East Side for another hour just to fuck with me. No sir, I had to play it cool. So after Tommy finished screaming at them through the driver's side window, trying to find out where they were taking me, I very nicely said, "Okay, it's just the three of us now. When we pull around the corner can you please stop and loosen these cuffs, they're seriously killing me. This is no joke."

"Oh, NOW you want to talk like a gentleman," said Ramos.

"I approached you like a gentleman from the beginning," I said. "I told you we were sorry and that my father is a retired sergeant, but your friend here decided to act like a douche-bag for some reason, so this is what happens. You can blame yourselves. Now I'm not kidding, you need to loosen these cuffs, there's no reason for them to be this tight. I've got no circulation in my hands right now."

"Take it easy, the station-house is only a few blocks away," said Ramos. That didn't stop him from taking the turns hard and fast just to toss me around a little.

When we pulled up to the station-house and they got me out of that tight little compartment where I was secretly freaking out, the two of them looked at each other as if to say, "Whoops, didn't we forgot something?" Then they started to pat me down and take everything out of my pockets as if that's what they meant to do all along.

"Shouldn't you guys have done this before you put me in the car?" I said. "What if I turned out to be some psychopath with a concealed weapon? That would have been bad for you guys, no?"

They didn't bother responding to that one.

Officer Fatfuck led me into the "house" like he had just made a major collar. "I bet your father never would've taken shit like that from anybody when he was a cop," he said in a very self-righteous way.

"My father never would have put himself in that position to begin with," I shot back. "That's the difference between a real cop and a crossing guard."

Poor Fatfuck. You could see the fight draining out of him.

Fortunately, when they toss you into the holding pen, they take the cuffs off. I had deep indents and cuts on both wrists and it took about twenty minutes for the life to come back into my hands, but the fight was starting to drain out of me at that point as well. I made a half-hearted attempt at intimidating the 17-year-old Puerto Rican kid who was in the holding cell with me because he had "borrowed" a couple of cell phones from two 12-year-olds, but I didn't carry it too far — the kid was scared shitless. I figured having to sit with me for an hour would be lesson enough.

Jimmy, Tommy, Billy and Matty found the precinct about half an hour later, but the cops wouldn't let them through the door until Matty ran into a detective he used to play softball with. Ramos came in to tell me it was my "lucky night," that the Sarge was in a "really good mood"

186

so they weren't going to take me downtown for processing after all.

"And this doesn't have anything to do with the fact that you never should have locked me up to begin with, does it?" I asked. Just to be clear.

For his part, Ramos left me with a summons for disorderly conduct. That's how he and Fatfuck were able to save face. And when I went down to the courthouse to pay the fine a few weeks later, admittedly a little nervous, it turned out that all the charges had been dropped.

Thus ended my fabulous 50th birthday and one-year-in-remission celebration, just me and the boys, Fatfuck and Ramos and a scared Puerto Rican kid. Good times.

You're probably wondering what the relevance of all of this is to my survivor story. Well, let me clear that up for you right quick: I never would have taken things that far with a cop to begin with had it not been for my chemically altered brain and that damn black cloud hanging over my head. And I wouldn't have a chemically altered brain or that damn black cloud if not for a year's worth of chemotherapy. And I wouldn't have had the chemo if not for that fucking cancer that found its way from my colon to my small intestine and lymph nodes. And I wouldn't have such a bad temper if not for the Sicilian blood flowing through my veins that was apparently supercharged by all that chemo. Ever since being pumped full of poison, I can no longer control my temper as well as I used to. Not to mention that John, one of my closest friends on the planet, was gone — wiped off the face of the fucking earth by that no good, miserable fucking Beast, and he was missing out on all the fun.

You see, it all makes perfect sense.

*

I never mentioned any of this to my family. If they do read this one day, it will take them by surprise. If I had to guess, Nick and Danny will think it's funny but that I'm a bit of an asshole; Brandon will think it's cool; Julianna will worry that I'm going to prison and she'll never see me again; Dana will worry that I'm not going to prison and she WILL see me again; and my father will give me one of those "angry cop" looks that even in my fifties still scares the shit out of me.

I can't wait! This is gonna make them all so proud!

Peace, Love, and Living in the Moment

Yeah, I wish.

I know there are a gazillion stories and books and blogs out there written by folks who have stumbled through the cancer labyrinth and made it to the other side relatively intact. Stories of hope, thanks, love, praise, support, and declarations to live every moment like it's their last. Awakenings, epiphanies, revelations and a-ha moments.

It's all fantastic. I truly hope that every one of those born-agains live long, happy, fulfilling lives.

But I have to tell you, I'm having a hell of a time feeling it three years into my remission. Don't get me wrong — I'm not the kind of guy who dwells in darkness. I'm actually very much the opposite. And I truly could not be happier to be surviving this fucked-up chapter of my life. I would love to remember how to experience every moment like an infant noticing a rainbow-colored blanket hanging over a crib for the first time, but it's not realistic. Who the fuck is actually fortunate enough to have nothing else to think about but how pretty a flower looks? Or how amazing it is when the sun breaks through the clouds after a rainstorm? I think the word most people use to describe a person like that is "simple." Boy, simple people have it made. And they don't even know it!

Puh-leeze. I've got so much shit floating around inside my head I can barely enjoy my morning pee, let alone the beauty of a field of wildflowers awakening to the fresh morning dew.

I can relate to what these people are talking about. I understand where all of this is coming from. When I was sick, when the odds were stacked against me — shit, yeah! Every moment counted. When I wasn't busy spitting on cancer and doing my best to squash it like a bug beneath my Timberlands, I took great delight in what normally would have been small moments.

I was particularly enamored of those moments involving my kids. I've always been very much tied into my children's lives — coaching their sports, walking them to school, talking them through whatever giant issue was at the top of their list, smothering them with affection (which makes Brandon crazy because he's 6-foot-3 now and thinks it's weird). I can't imagine what a blow it would have been to them if I suddenly disappeared. Or to Dana. Or to my parents. My brother and sisters. My friends. Christ.

As you now know, I've lost several close friends to the disease while I was in the middle of my "journey." (Doesn't that word make the whole thing sound magical?) I know what it does to someone who cares about you when you close your eyes for the last time. This is the one thing that weighed on me most heavily. The prospect of death itself was a distant second.

I'm not very religious, but I have always considered myself to be spiritual. I have very strong beliefs in a higher entity and in the eternal validity of the soul (which will be available for you to read in more detail once our "what do you think happens when you die" findings are published. I'm just waiting for John to reach out and give me some additional insight from the other side). So I'm really not afraid of dying. And if I'm wrong, so what? There's not a damn thing any of us can do about what happens once we've shuffled off this mortal coil. It's living that's difficult. It takes every bit of energy just to keep the train on the tracks, never mind moving in the right direction.

But I digress.

One of my favorite authors, Tom Robbins, wrote a stanza in his masterful novel *Still Life With Woodpecker* that has stayed with me ever since I first read it in college:

"There is only one serious question. And that is: *Who knows how to make love stay?* Answer me that and I will tell you whether or not to kill yourself. Answer me that and I will ease your mind about the beginning and the end of time. Answer me that and I will reveal to you the purpose of the moon."

Well, I'm sorry to contradict you Tom, but I have learned through experience that there are actually two serious questions. And while it would be impossible to top the first one, I respectfully propose this as a follow-up:

Who knows how to make that blissful feeling of "living in the moment" stay?

Shit, answer me that and I'll ...

But back to my point. Yes, I can relate to what those folks are talking about because I caught a fleeting glimpse of it myself. It was spectacular. Time slowed to a crawl and I was at peace with the world. It was absolutely amazing. But then somebody handed me back the reins and "real" life came crashing back in — the one where I'm the control freak who has to do everything himself because everything has to be done a certain way and I'm the only one who knows how to do it; the one where I'll never be able to forget that I had Stage IV colon cancer as I ponder how long miracles actually last; the one where bills still need to be paid and the kids are screaming and Dana is freaking out and work sucks. In other words, the life I only felt comfortable taking my eye off because I had no choice. To get well again, I needed to focus on nothing but getting well, and that meant letting others pick up the slack for me, or what I imagined was slack that needed picking up.

But, hey — that's life. Real life. And we're all in it together.

I was lucky to experience "tuning out" for that brief period. It was incredibly liberating. I could have announced to the world that I intended to think about nothing but butterflies on a particular day, so please do not disturb. I could have spent an entire week mulling over butterflies if I so chose. Interaction with real-life concerns was temporarily suspended whenever I needed it to be; all I had to do was pull out the cancer card, tears welling: "Thinking about butterflies really helps me deal with my cancer and handle the chemo."

While I wouldn't recommend getting cancer as a way of having the unmitigated freedom of engaging in such absurdity, I have to say I learned a lot about myself from it. I'm still amazed that I was able to endure having my entire abdomen marinated in poison for three months. For that alone, I should get a free pass (along with everyone else who has ever gone through HIPEC or EPIC). In retrospect, that's the one thing I'm really proud of myself for (notwithstanding my new-found appreciation of Danaus plexippus). Toughing it out through the most demanding aspect of my physical recovery was a genuine achievement. This was one of those rare opportunities where the decision you make and the approach you take can mean the difference between life and, well, non-life (you see what I mean about that "non" thing; now it's back to being bad). It was like winning an Iron Man competition when my training consisted of playing a little softball and running across the street to avoid oncoming traffic. I know in what's left of my gut that this is the thing that gave me the edge I needed over the Beast.

"They really put you through hell," Dr. Fuks was kind enough to tell me recently. "I would never want to go through what you went through. You should give yourself a lot of credit, my friend. You contributed as much to your own recovery as your doctors did. Without a strong desire, it's very difficult to handle something like this. You were very determined right from the beginning." Cancer? Puhh!!

From time to time, I am now able to consciously slow things down and be in the moment, but only for a moment. It's not something I was able to do before I got sick because it takes a ton of concentration. I guess that's why so many people love to meditate. Me, I find it easier to medicate. Takes less patience.

Okay, so maybe I haven't emerged from my travels "born again" into a life where I unquestioningly appreciate all things, smile and sing pretty songs, while I forgive and forget. So what? It's an unreasonable expectation of anyone.

The thing I hear most often from people when they become aware of what I went through is, "Wow, you must have a completely different perspective on life now." I get it, but I really wish they'd stop. I certainly viewed things differently while in the heat of battle, but I no longer have that luxury. Real life doesn't change or go away, it hides around the corner and waits. When you're back inside it, it's scary and lonely and loving and hateful and exciting and boring and stressful and peaceful and hectic and completely unpredictable, and I'm okay with that. I'm okay with all of it.

But I do miss being spoiled. When I finally gave in and allowed myself to be treated "special" by everyone,

194

that special attention so outweighed the horrors of surgery and treatment and all the rest that I almost didn't want to get better. I know that sounds fucking nuts, but it's true. I let myself get spoiled. And I liked it. And it left me completely unprepared for what it would be like to re-enter real life, post-cancer.

The woods are lovely, dark and deep.
But I have promises to keep,
And miles to go before I sleep,
And miles to go before I sleep.

"Stopping By Woods on a Snowy Evening" — Robert Frost

Epilogue:
Wise Master, Share With Us What You Have Learned On Your Journey

Well, let me see, my worthy friends. What have I learned on my journey? I must say that your hunger for knowledge inspires me, and your thirst for truth fills my heart with great joy. I offer you now the following tidbits and encourage you to share them with others who may hunger for knowledge and thirst for truth (or may just be curious about what a man who was mighty, mighty sick but got better has to say):

For starters, I guess it's fair to say that in spite of the fact that my life is still stressful and challenging (whose isn't?), and I don't open my eyes each morning and view the world with the wonder of a child (who does?), one thing has become quite clear: It's good to be alive. Yes, sir, I've taken an unexpectedly close look at the alternative and I'm here to tell you, it's fucking good to be alive.

Here's a biggie: Phase II of the recovery process, the emotional and psychological recovery, can be more difficult than Phase I, the physical recovery. It was and still is for me. It's so important to know this because you have to be ready for it. You need time to prepare. It hit me like a ton of bricks as I was bending down to tie my shoe. I never saw it coming.

How about this one: Fear of the unknown can be far more debilitating than walking right up and waltzing with whatever beast or demon stands in your way. Fear of the unknown begets anxiety, and anxiety wreaks havoc on your brain's ability to process and make sense of things. Being anxious about the what if's is far more stressful and incapacitating than actually knowing what's wrong — even if, as in my case, what's wrong is heavily weighted toward the Big Sleep side of the scale. Here's the thing: Wrapping my brain around it and understanding the details and treatment options set me on the path to recovery. There was a plan in place. We (me, Zvi, my doctors, my family and friends) were taking action, and taking action is in and of itself very empowering.

Let me say that one more time, and you should write it down: Taking action is in and of itself very empowering. Don't just stand there, do something. Anything. You'll start to feel better about things the moment you do.

Here's another one: I'm really a lucky bastard. When I was diagnosed in August 2007, the Beast was already active not only in my upper colon, but on my small intestine and in my lymph nodes as well. Freak cells at Stage IV. It was seeding my abdomen with its nasty little clones. Holy shit! I know it doesn't sound like it, but I am very lucky. Glass half full beats glass half empty every time.

This one is very important: I've come to realize that no matter how hopeless or dire the situation, nothing is inevitable. Miracles occur all the time. I know, because I'm one of them. And I'm not alone. I know a bunch of other miracles, too. Personal friends. Armed with this knowledge, it is essential that you let the potential for a miracle keep driving you forward.

You probably already know this, but I'm going to say it anyway: Support is a key component of your recovery. What you probably don't realize is that support is also key for the people who care about you. Share the load. Your family, friends and colleagues are all affected by your diagnosis. They need to understand what you're going through so they can take action and be empowered as well. They need to support you because, through no fault of their own, support is the only thing they can contribute to your battle. They need to help you get better so that *they* can get better. Sharing the load also seems to sap the Beast's strength, which is a good thing.

Now hear this: The "power of positive thinking" isn't some hokey, New-Age hippie catchphrase born of taking one toke too many; it's for real. Positive energy heals. Whether you're religious or spiritual or nothing at all, put positive thoughts and energy out there. In my experience, it seems to help. It sure doesn't hurt.

This one seems so obvious, but it eluded me: Listen to your body. It knows when something's not right and it sends you messages in the form of pain and discomfort. Don't always assume things will go away on their own if you just ignore them. If your gut (no pun intended) tells you that you should pay attention, pay attention.

Short & Sweet: Don't be foolish enough to count on luck to get you through life, because luck is a fickle friend. *Make your own shit happen.*

You may or may not believe this one, but I know for a fact that angels hang out on 68th Street and York Avenue in New York City. I kid you not. It's been my observation that when angels come down to earth, they gather at a little club called Memorial Sloan-Kettering Cancer Center. They must be angels to do what they do every day with a smile and an encouraging word always at the ready. Angels on 68th Street. Isn't that a movie? It should be.

Friends. Yes, indeed, friends. As Elton John and Bernie Taupin were kind enough to remind us: *With a friend at hand, you will see the light / If your friends are there, then everything's all right.* I can't imagine where I'd be right now if not for my friends, and I don't restrict that sentiment to cancer recovery.

Survivor guilt. Whew, this one really throws you for a loop. It's devastating to tell someone who has lost a loved one to the disease that you are now cancer free and doing fine. You feel as though you've betrayed the deceased in some way. You can't understand how you survived while someone else, possibly your closest friend, didn't. Get help if you ever find yourself in this situation. It will take a long, long time to come to terms with this. I'm still working on it.

I'd love to be able to share with you how to live in the moment and appreciate life to its fullest, but I can't, because I have no fucking idea how to do that. I'm much too preoccupied with how I'm gonna pay the bills at the end of each month and how I'm gonna keep my children safe and sound. Someone else is going to have to fill you in on the secrets of LITM. But I can tell you this: You should make it your business to ensure that the people you care about know how you feel about them at all times. Don't take it for granted. It only takes a moment to show or tell someone how much they mean to you. Put the petty shit aside and make amends because when life sly-raps you or your loved one in the back of the head one day, you'll regret not having your affairs in order. And regret is a motherfucker.

And finally, if the Beast shows up unexpectedly at your door one day, you need to go at it head on. Go strong, straight out of the gate. Kick the bastard in the balls. Showing the sonofabitch the slightest bit of fear or deference only serves to make it meaner and more powerful. Don't cower and don't be afraid — be disrespectful. Look that Beast in the eye and say what Walter would have said: "Puhh! Fuck you!" I'm not saying it's easy, because it's not. But it is do-able. I've said it before and I'll say it again — it's amazing what we're capable of when our backs are to the wall and we're about to get slammed.

Never give up, and never give in.

Spit instead.

Spit a lot.

Cancer? Please.

To quote Matthew (1:1) -

"Puhh!! That's your mother in there!"

Author's Note

For the record, I mean no disrespect to the New York City Police Department. In fact, I have nothing but respect for it as an organization. I think I just bumped into a couple of guys who were in a shitty mood themselves that random Thursday night in August and one thing led to another and, pretty soon ... Ahh, never mind; scratch that. Those two guys were assholes.

The events in this book are true and accurate to the best of my recollection. My intent is not to downplay the seriousness of cancer, but to demystify diagnosis and treatment, raise awareness, offer encouragement, and let the reader know that it is possible to continue with life while limping down the long and winding road to recovery.

If you're supporting a friend or relative who is going through the drill, support that person with humor and do your best to bring normalcy to the party. Learn to read the signs: Sometimes the person will want company, sometimes not. Sometimes he or she may need to talk through some serious issues; other times they'll just want to veg out watching a movie and laugh. Distract them with nonsense. Don't take their mood swings personally. Bring them food and make them eat it. Take over the college tuition or mortgage payments for a year or two (not a requirement, but an incredibly nice gesture).

Any and all explanations of medical procedures and treatments of cancer in this book, including surgery and systemic / intraperitoneal chemotherapy, represent my understanding of such procedures and treatments only. I have no medical training or education whatsoever, so please don't quote me or use this book as a substitute for a medical opinion.

Any derogatory references made herein to friends, or to acquaintances who were on the verge of becoming friends, are made out of love and affection and are intended to be humorous. I don't want anybody calling me up with big bitch tears saying stuff like, "How could you write something like that about me? I thought we were friends." We *are* friends. I'm just capitalizing on an opportunity to be funny at your expense.

203

Acknowledgments

My wife and children, who make it all worthwhile (sometimes — OK, a lot of the time. — alright, most of the time); my father, who has never failed to show me by way of example what it is to be a good parent, a good friend, and a good man; my brother and sisters and all my wonderful in-laws, nieces and nephews who helped me stand on my own two feet when the weight of the world decided to take rest upon my shoulders (fucking weight of the world — Puhh!); Jami Bernard, without whom you never would have read this story (if you're a writer or wish to be one, Google her — you won't regret it); Jon Robson, Benny Battista, Ed Miller and all my friends and colleagues at TR who removed confusion and anxiety from the equation and allowed me to focus on getting well again; Zvi Fuks, Jose, David, Steve, and all the angels and saints at MSKCC (Amen to that); Ed Renehan, who was crazy and sweet enough to publish this story; and, finally, the Beast, whom I hate with all my heart, but whom I must acknowledge has taught me some important lessons about life, love and the pursuit of happiness (but still — Puhh!).

About the Author

James Capuano is Senior Vice President for the Markets Division of Thomas Reuters, the global news and information company. He lives in Manhattan with his wife Dana and their four children.

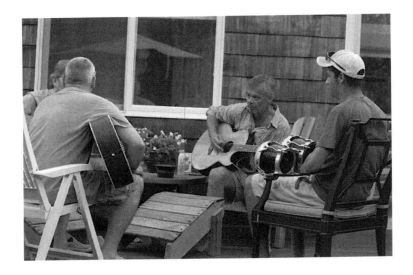

Capuano and friends, Fire Island, 2012.

205

About the Publisher

New Street Communications, LLC, publishes and distributes superior works of nonfiction (and, through our Dark Hall Press imprint, select fiction in the Horror genre). We are a *digital-native* imprint. As such, we primarily make our titles available as eBooks, though often in paper editions as well. On the nonfiction side of things, we cover the intersection of digital technology and society; transformative business communication and innovation (particularly the conceptualizing of elegant new tools, markets, products and paradigms); socially-relevant children's literature; and literary criticism. New Street's nonfiction books are authored by distinguished scholars, journalists, entrepreneurs, developers and thought leaders.

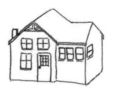

newstreetcommunications.com

Made in the USA
San Bernardino, CA
10 December 2013

6485849R00118